QUALITY OF LIFE

FOR PEOPLE WITH INTELLECTUAL AND
OTHER DEVELOPMENTAL DISABILITIES

APPLICATIONS ACROSS INDIVIDUALS, ORGANIZATIONS, COMMUNITIES, AND SYSTEMS

QUALITY OF LIFE

FOR PEOPLE WITH INTELLECTUAL AND OTHER DEVELOPMENTAL DISABILITIES

APPLICATIONS ACROSS INDIVIDUALS, ORGANIZATIONS, COMMUNITIES, AND SYSTEMS

ROBERT L. SCHALOCK

JAMES F. GARDNER

VALERIE J. BRADLEY

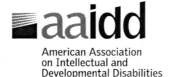

American Association
on Intellectual and
Developmental Disabilities

Published by
American Association on Intellectual and Developmental Disabilities
444 North Capitol Street, NW
Suite 846
Washington, DC 20001-1512

Printed in the United States of America

Library of Congress Cataloging-in-Publication Data

Schalock, Robert L.
Quality of life for persons with intellectual and other developmental
disabilities : applications across individuals, organizations,
communities, and systems / Robert L. Schalock, James F. Gardner, Valerie
J. Bradley.
        p. ; cm.
    Includes bibliographical references and index.
    ISBN 0-940898-96-9
    1. Developmentally disabled. 2. People with mental disabilities--Rehabilita-
tion. 3. People with disabilities--Rehabilitation. 4. Quality of life. I. Gardner, James
F., 1946- II. Bradley, Valerie J. III. American Association on Intellectual and Developmental Disabilities. IV. Title.
    HV1570.S335 2007
    362.4'0458--dc22
                                                      2007008026

Table of Contents

List of Tables v

List of Figures vii

Preface ix

Part 1: The Individual Perspective 1

Chapter 1. The Concepts of Quality of Life and Personal Outcomes 3

Chapter 2. Quality Domains and Indicators 15

Chapter 3. Measuring Personal Outcomes: An Information Collection Process 29

Part 2: The Organizational Perspective 45

Chapter 4. Managerial Strategies: Opening the Doors Inward 47

Chapter 5. Personal Outcome Measures: Values and Metrics for an Integrated

Management System 71

Part 3: The Systems Perspective 93

Chapter 6. Rationale for Systems-Level Performance Indicators That Reflect

Personal Outcomes 97

Chapter 7. Considerations in Developing Performance Indicators at the Macro Level 109

Chapter 8. How Do I Use Performance Indicator Data? 129

Part 4: Quality of Life for People With Intellectual and Other Developmental

Disabilities: Going Forward 143

Chapter 9. Reframing Quality and Rethinking Quality Improvement 147

Chapter 10. Emerging Challenges and Opportunities 169

References 181

Subject Index 197

List of Tables

Table 1.1. Quality of Life Conceptualization, Measurement, and Application Principles 6

Table 1.2. Guidelines for Using Personal Outcomes for Personal Development, Personal Well-Being, and Quality Improvement 7

Table 1.3. Quality of Life Domains and Quality Indicators 9

Table 2.1. Changing Approaches to Accountability 16

Table 2.2. Five Useful Purposes of Quality Indicators 17

Table 2.3. Quality Factors: Content Analysis of Individual-Referenced Domains 20

Table 2.4. Quality of Life Domains and Associated Quality Indicators 21

Table 2.5. Personal Outcome Measures and Associated Quality Indicators 22

Table 2.6. Core Domains and Associated Quality Indicators 23

Table 2.7. Commonly Referenced Investigators and Respective Quality Domains and Indicators 25

Table 2.8. Criteria for Selecting Quality Indicators 27

Table 3.1. Principles Underlying the Measurement of Quality Outcomes 31

Table 3.2. Guidelines for Collecting Quality of Life Information 33

Table 3.3. Psychometric Standards Governing the Measurement of Personal Outcomes 36

Table 3.4. Suggestions for Overcoming Measurement Challenges and Potential Resistance 41

Table 4.1. Outcome Design Index™ 55

Table 5.1. Summary of Data on Personal Measurement Outcomes and Organizational Supports Collected Nationwide During Accreditation Reviews 80

Table 5.2. Sample Benchmarking and Comparison Data for Alpha, Inc. 82

Table 5.3. Predictions of Quality of Life and Accreditation Outcomes 85

Table 5.4. Outcomes That Predict Achieving the Largest Number of Outcomes 86

Table 7.1. Percentage of Respondents Answering "Yes" to National Core Indicators 111

Table 7.2. Potential Performance Indicators That Reflect Personal Outcomes 114

Table 7.3. Death Rate Among People With ID-DD in Massachusetts Compared With General Population 126

Table 8.1. Crosswalk of National Core Indicators Data Sources to CMS Quality Framework 131

Table 8.2. Comparison of Consumer Outcomes: Rhode Island Quality Consortium 136

Table 9.1. Strategies Characterizing a "Reframing Quality" and "Rethinking Quality Improvement" Mental Model 157

Table 9.2. Key Leadership Themes That Facilitate Personal Outcomes 167

Lists of Figures

Figure 1.1. Operationalizing the quality of life construct: Domains and indicators 8

Figure 3.1. Effectiveness of proxies to measure personal outcomes and support needs 37

Figure 4.1. Organizational factors that enhance personal outcomes 50

Figure 4.2. Quality of life strategy initiatives 52

Figure 4.3. Function of quality leadership in a service-based organization 65

Figure 5.1. Integrated quality system for an organization providing disability services 72

Figure 6.1. Factors influencing the need for systems-level performance indicators 98

Figure 6.2. U.S. Centers for Medicare and Medicaid Services, quality framework for home and community-based services 105

Figure 7.1. Percentage of individual respondents indicating case manager helps get what person needs 124

Figure 7.2. Percentage of respondents who went to the dentist in the past six months 125

Figure 7.3. Longitudinal comparison of family perceptions of effectiveness of case managers 127

Figure 8.1. Percentage of people experiencing respectful interactions with staff 134

Figure 8.2. National Core Indicators consumer survey: Year-to-year comparsion— relationships 138

Figure 9.1. Integrated systems thinking 151

Figure 9.2. Symbols involved in reframing quality and rethinking quality improvement 163

Figure 9.3. Changing relationships among organizations, people, and community 164

Figure 9.4. Relationships to be explored among organizations, people, and community 166

Figure 10.1. Quality-improvement process 178

PREFACE

This book is about the quality of life of people with intellectual and other developmental disabilities (ID-DD). It's also about how to conceptualize, measure, and apply the quality of life (QOL) construct to enhance their lives. Historically the QOL concept has been used primarily as a sensitizing notion that during the 1980s and 1990s grounded and guided what an individual valued and desired. During the past decade, its role has expanded to include: (a) a conceptual framework for assessing personal outcomes, (b) a social construct that guides quality improvement strategies, and (c) a criterion for assessing the effectiveness of those strategies. As such, it has become an agent for social change that at its core makes us think differently about people with ID-DD and how we might reform policy and practice to enhance personal outcomes.

The initial idea for this book came from a May 2002 American Association on Mental Retardation (AAMR) preconference workshop titled Quality Indicators and Performance Measures: Can We Get on the Same Page? The workshop focused on (a) the changing quality landscape; (b) the evolving need for service providers, funders, and policy makers to employ an integrated approach to quality outcomes and their use for people with ID-DD; and (c) the emerging development of data-based internal quality improvement mechanisms.

Since then, it has become increasingly clear that the large-scale adoption of a person-centered approach to basic assurances and QOL assessment requires a data-driven quality model. Unfortunately those who search for such a model confront a seeming paradox. As discussed by Gardner and Carran (2005),

> The traditional standards and methods associated with procedural compliance and documentation are, by themselves, insufficient to address the variables that impact quality supports and quality of life of people. At the same time, we have not yet succeeded in developing a new quality

assessment and improvement methodology grounded in person-centered assurances and quality of life assessment. (p. 158)

This book, which addresses the needed quality assessment and improvement process, presents a data-driven quality model that reflects our current thinking and best practices regarding the understanding and use of the QOL concept across individuals, organizations, communities, and systems. The book has five objectives:

1. To rethink what is meant by quality of life and how the QOL concept has become a change agent. In that regard, we link various developments in the field of ID-DD to the evolution of the QOL concept and its use.

2. To synthesize current research and literature on quality of life and its measurement and discuss how the concept has influenced management strategies, organizational design, systems change, and leadership. We do this within the context of community networks of resources and supports.

3. To provide examples of how the QOL concept can be operationalized, measured, and applied at the individual, organizational, and systems levels. In this process, we (a) present a set of criteria and guidelines regarding its conceptualization, measurement, and application, and (b) discuss how QOL-related information can be integrated at the individual, organizational, and systems level.

4. To show how QOL-related information can be used in an intentional way to enhance personal outcomes. In the process, we illustrate factors external to our field that influence how we do business and how we measure performance.

5. To move beyond traditional terms and concepts (e.g., standards, program-specific requirements, process measurement, and quality as compliance) to a QOL focus with its emphasis on the achievement of personal outcomes. To that end, we discuss challenges and opportunities and suggest positive ways to address them.

In writing the book, we have kept in mind our readers' perspectives. Although we anticipate our primary readers to be service providers and policy makers, we also expect people with disabilities, public-sector funders, training personnel, and graduate students in training programs to find the book valuable. To one degree or another, over the past decade all of these stakeholder groups have experienced significant changes in terms of services and supports, including: (a) advancing person-centered supports and self-determination, (b) emphasizing quality outcomes in addition to quality processes, (c) recognizing the changes in experiences and expectations of people with disabilities and their families, (d) moving away from prescriptive standards, (e) emphasizing quality (i.e., continuous) improvement, and (f) involving people with disabilities in the design, delivery, and evaluation of services and supports.

Of course changes are also occurring at societal levels, including: (a) a transformed vision of what constitutes the life possibilities of people with ID-DD, including an emphasis on self-determination, community inclusion, equity, and human potential; (b) an ecological conception of disability that focuses on the person and the environment; (c) the development of community-based options and support systems; (d) the implementation of service options, including the direct purchase of services and supports; (e) the use of the QOL concept as a basis for best practices; (f) the emergence of the reform movement with its emphasis on measurability, reportability, and accountability; and (g) the use of QOL-related outcome information for multiple purposes, including increasing the transparency of systems through the dissemination of information, improving services and supports, and guiding the change process. These changes reflect the need for a book that presents a quality assessment and improvement methodology grounded in person-centered assurances and QOL assessment.

Book Organization

The book discusses the perspectives of the individual (part 1), the organization (part 2), and the larger system (part 3).

In part 1 we introduce the concept of quality of life and personal outcomes, the use of quality indicators to operationalize these outcomes, and the measurement strategies and guidelines used in QOL assessment. This section provides the conceptual basis for the development and use of personal outcomes as well as the challenges involved in moving from individual data collection and analysis to the complexities involved in data aggregation and use at the organizational and systems level. Although focusing primarily on *person-centered QOL domains and indicators*, the concepts, principles, and practices also apply to families and their quality of life. For a detailed discussion of current work in the area of family quality of life, see Poston et al. (2003) and Summers et al. (2005).

Part 2 is focused primarily on management strategies that open organizational doors inward to enable people to understand their own strengths and unique capabilities that integrate values, people, and measurement. Part 2 also explores the emerging trends in the measurement and use of personal outcomes within the context of community-oriented applications of personal quality of life.

Part 3 discusses the rationale for systems-level performance indicators that reflect personal outcomes. Within that context, we discuss how one might think about and approach the development of performance indicators and how systems can use performance data to enhance the provision of services and supports.

The book concludes with a "going forward" discussion of the need to (a) reframe quality and rethink quality improvement, and (b) embrace a number of important challenges and opportunities.

Defining Terms

Right up front we want to define some important terms used throughout the book. Although there are slight variations in meaning depending on the focus (i.e., individual, organizational, or systems), their general definitions are as follows:

- *Personal outcomes*: Person-defined and valued aspirations. Personal outcomes are generally defined in reference to QOL domains and indicators. They can be (a) analyzed at the level of the individual, (b) aggregated at the provider and/or systems level, and/or (c) complemented by other systems-level indicators (e.g., health and safety indicators, staff turnover, membership on community boards).

- *Quality of life domains*: The set of factors comprising personal well-being. The set represents the range over which the QOL concept extends and thus defines quality of life.

- *Quality indicators*: QOL-related perceptions, behaviors, and conditions that give an indication of a person's well-being.

- *Performance indicators*: A comprehensive set of indicators at the organizational or systems level that typically includes: (a) aggregated quality indicators, and (b) other indicators, such as staff turnover, annual medical and dental examinations, mortality rates, incident or injury rate.

- *Quality improvement*: An organization's or a system's capacity to improve performance and accountability through systematically collecting and analyzing data and information and implementing action strategies based on the analysis. Its goal is to improve the quality of life of individuals by enhancing policies, practices, training, technical assistance, and other organizational- and/or systems-level supports.

- *Intellectual disabilities*: Term that refers to individuals who manifest developmentally related significant limitations in both intellectual functioning and adaptive behavior as expressed in conceptual, social, and practical adaptive skills. Commonly used synonyms are *mental retardation* and *cognitive disabilities*.

- *Developmental disabilities*: A number of developmentally related impairment groups and diagnostic conditions that include: (a) cognitive impairments, such as metabolic and immune deficiency disorders and chromosomal abnormalities; (b) sensory-neurological impairments, such as epilepsy and spina bifida; (c) physical impairments, such as cerebral palsy; and (d) emotional-behavioral impairments, such as autism or dual diagnosis.

The book is based on our 110 years of collective experience in the field of ID-DD. It represents our best attempt to synthesize what we currently know about best practices related to the QOL concept and its use at the individual, organizational, and systems levels. In writing a book on quality of life and personal outcomes, one challenge involves defining *quality* and answering the question, "What is the quality in quality?" Most definitions of *quality* include terms such as *essential character,* an *inherent feature,* or a *distinguishing attribute.* What's more, to both service recipients and agency- and systems-level personnel, *quality* means desired attributes of services and supports and valued, personal outcomes. Throughout the book, we use the term *quality* to refer to both (a) the process through which services and supports are provided to individuals with ID-DD, and (b) a valued, personal outcome from those services.

In the end this book is a journey that begins with determining what is important in people's lives and then developing the services and supports that enhance personal outcomes reflecting a person's hopes and dreams. It is a journey that begins with the concept of quality of life and progresses to its implementation at the individual, organizational, community, and systems level.

Acknowledgments

Some of the material in this book is taken from work previously published and copyrighted by the Council on Quality and Leadership (parts 2 and 3). We also acknowledge the significant work that numerous states have devoted to the development of the National Core Indicators (part 3).

The book could not have been written without some "help from our friends." Our personal appreciation to those consumers, program personnel, policy makers, and colleagues who have assisted us in that journey by providing insight, inspiration, and guidance. A very special thank you as well to Darlene Buschow, who provided technical support and encouragement throughout our writing and editing.

Robert L. Schalock
James F. Gardner
Valerie J. Bradley
January 2007

PART 1

The Individual Perspective

Personal outcomes for people with intellectual and other developmental disabilities (ID-DD) are embedded within the quality of life (QOL) concept. Thus our journey begins with (a) an in-depth discussion of the QOL construct and the significant impact it has had on the development and evaluation of services and supports to people with disabilities, and (b) the evidence-based management strategies that accompany its implementation.

This section introduces individual-referenced quality of life and how it can be conceptualized and measured through the assessment of quality indicators. Over the past three decades, the QOL construct has provided the conceptual basis for quality outcomes and their application; it has become increasingly important as a *sensitizing notion* that gives reference and guidance from the individual's perspective, a *conceptual framework* for assessing quality outcomes, a *social construct* that guides program enhancement strategies, and a *criterion for assessing* the effectiveness of those strategies. This evolution is reflected in how we conceptualize and measure the construct and how it is applied at the organizational (part 2) and systems (part 3) levels.

The following three chapters and the guidelines presented therein rely on a sequential thought process that begins with a model that establishes parameters to how one conceptualizes quality and then provides a framework for developing quality indicators. The measurement of those quality indicators results in personal outcomes.

Part 1 focuses on quality of life and how we approach its conceptualization and measurement. In that regard, chapter 1 describes the key role the QOL concept plays in personal outcomes, reviews the concept's recent history, and distinguishes personal outcomes from social indicators. Material in this chapter also relates changes in evaluation theory to our approach to the measurement and use of personal outcomes.

QOL conceptualization and measurement pose at least two challenges, relating to issues raised in chapter 2: (a) by definition, the evaluation of quality is subjective and therefore nonprescriptive, so (b) how does one take the subjective, somewhat amorphous concept and make it measurable? Chapter 2 addresses these two challenges and discusses the need to operationalize quality of life into its respective domains and measurable indicators. The majority of chapter 2 is devoted to a literature-based summary of the most commonly used QOL models and their respective domains and indicators. The chapter also discusses the context and use of quality indicators and the key role they play in establishing personal outcomes for people with ID-DD. The chapter concludes with a discussion of 10 criteria for selecting a set of quality indicators to serve as the basis for the measurement of personal outcomes. These criteria represent a delicate balance between person-defined and valued QOL aspirations and program-driven quality indicators. As discussed in chapters 2, 4, and 5, we are slowly making the transition from program-driven quality indicators to indicators that are personally defined and driven (i.e., personal goals and aspirations).

Personal outcomes and their measurement are the focus of chapter 3. The chapter begins with a general discussion of the value of measuring personal outcomes and four principles that should guide their measurement. The chapter then summarizes an information collection process based on two components: (a) an in-person interview that identifies valued personal outcomes, and (b) a discrepancy analysis conducted by placing the person within the context of community indicators. As discussed later in the text, the purpose of quality improvement is to reduce the discrepancy between valued personal outcomes and community indicators. The chapter then outlines strategies for using the proposed information collection process to measure personal outcomes, and it concludes with an example of how to progress from measuring personal outcomes to using that data for quality improvement. Chapter 3 makes the important point that although personal outcomes can be used for multiple purposes, their assessment is made at the level of the individual.

Keep the following four QOL conceptualization principles clearly in mind as you read part 1: quality of life (a) is multidimensional and influenced by personal and environmental factors and their interactions, (b) has the same components for all people, (c) has both subjective and objective components, and (d) is enhanced by self-determination, resources, purpose in life, and a sense of belonging.

The intent of chapters 1–3 is to provide the reader with a better understanding of the QOL concept from the individual's perspective and establish a basis for its measurement and application. In that regard, keep the following four points in mind: (a) Although quality is nonprescriptive, individuals, organizations, and systems-level personnel need a clear understanding of QOL domains and indicators in order to implement an integrated approach to the evaluation of personal outcomes; (b) this integrated approach should be grounded in what we currently know about the QOL concept and its measurement; (c) the structure and content of any outcome measurement system needs to fit its intended use and philosophical foundation; and (d) the conceptual framework and integrated approach outlined provides a number of stakeholder benefits including a common language and information that can be used to enhance valued outcomes, improve management strategies, and guide judgments.

CHAPTER 1

The Concepts of Quality of Life and Personal Outcomes

Introduction and Overview

Our discussion of personal outcomes for people with intellectual disabilities and other developmental disabilities (ID-DD) begins with the concept of quality of life. The purpose of this chapter is to review the recent history of the quality of life (QOL) concept and describe how it has emerged at the level of the individual as the basis for assessing personal outcomes.

At its core the QOL concept makes us think differently about people at the margin of society and how we might bring about change at the organizational, systems, and community levels to enhance people's personal well-being and to reduce their exclusion from the societal mainstream. Quality of life is a multidimensional concept that includes a number of domains that reflect positive values and life experiences. Although these domains are sensitive to cultural and life-span perspectives, they typically involve desired states related to personal well-being. The QOL concept is important because it is

- a sensitizing notion that gives us reference and guidance from the individual's perspective, focusing on the core domains of a life of quality;

- a conceptual framework for assessing quality outcomes;

- a social construct that guides performance enhancement strategies;

- a criterion for assessing the effectiveness of those strategies.

In today's human service programs, quality is pursued at three levels: (a) people who desire a life of quality, (b) providers who want to deliver a product that results in enhanced personal outcomes, and (c) policy makers and funders who desire valued outcomes for service recipients and data that can link services and supports to these outcomes. This emphasis on quality of life also reflects (a) a transformed vision of what constitutes the life possibilities of people with ID-DD; (b) a new way of thinking about people with ID-DD that focuses on the person, the environmental variables that influence the person's functioning, and the feasibility of change at individual, organizational, and systems levels; (c) the current paradigm shift with its emphasis on inclusion, equity, empowerment, and community-based supports; and (d) the quality revolution with its emphasis on quality improvement and valued person-referenced outcomes.

Rather than defining quality of life (there are more than 100 definitions in the literature), we set the stage for this book by (a) summarizing the evolution and impact of the QOL construct, (b) making a distinction between social indicators and personal outcomes, and (c) relating changes in evaluation theory to our approach to the measurement and use of quality indicators and personal outcomes. Although the primary focus of the chapter is the individual, we will refer, where appropriate, to the organization and the larger system within which individuals and organizations implement the QOL concept.

Quality of Life Over Three Decades

The QOL concept is not new, for a discussion of what constitutes well-being and happiness dates back to Plato and Aristotle. Yet over the past three decades, the concept has become a primary focus of person-centered planning, outcome evaluation, and quality improvement (Schalock, 2004; Schalock & Verdugo, 2002). To appreciate fully the importance of this concept and its recent history, it is necessary to understand its semantic meaning, which also explains its emergence as a sensitizing notion, a conceptual framework, a social construct, and a criterion to evaluate the validity and effectiveness of quality improvement strategies. In reference to its meaning, *quality* makes us think of the excellence or "exquisite standard" associated with human characteristics and positive values, such as happiness and satisfaction; *of life* indicates that the concept concerns the very essence or essential aspects of human existence. Although this semantic meaning has remained the same over the past three decades, the understanding and use of the concept has evolved.

The 1980s
Throughout much of the world, the 1980s was a time of the quality revolution and opportunity development. In the United States, for example, legislation focused on quality and opportunities through the passage of numerous federal statutes and the enactment of federal and state court decisions (Turnbull, Wilcox, Stowe, & Umbarger, 2001). Advocacy was also advanced during this decade through the founding of Disabled Peoples International in Singapore and the United Nations proclaiming 1981 as the International Year of Disabled Persons (Hayden & Nelis, 2002).

The field of ID-DD embraced the QOL concept during the 1980s primarily for four reasons. First, it captured the changing views of people with disabilities as reflected in self-determination, inclusion, empowerment, and equity. Thus during the 1980s, the QOL concept captured the changing vision and became the vehicle through which consumer-referenced equity, empowerment, and increased life satisfaction could be achieved. Second, it provided a common language that reflected the goals of normalization, deinstitutionalization, and mainstreaming and also met the need for program accountability. Third, it was consistent with the quality revolution, with its emphasis on quality products and quality outcomes. Thus the QOL concept was applied to human service programs and thereby integrated person-centered planning, the supports model, personal outcomes, and quality improvement. Fourth, it reflected the expectations among recipients that the services and supports they receive will significantly and positively influence their personal well-being.

The 1990s

In the field of ID-DD, the 1990s saw accelerated change and adjustment, a rethinking and redrafting of policies. The Americans With Disabilities Act of 1990, the reauthorization of the Individuals With Disabilities Education Act of 1991, and the 1992 Rehabilitation Act Amendments comprised a body of antidiscrimination legislation and service priorities that emphasized greater access to services and full involvement of individuals with disabilities in community life and service delivery. At the same time, education and rehabilitation programs were being influenced by the reform movement with its focus on quality, accountability, and outputs rather than inputs (Schalock, 2001).

The quality revolution of the 1980s, with its emphasis on quality of life and opportunity development, merged with the reform movement of the 1990s, with its focus on quality outcomes and accountability. The net result? The QOL construct was thrust into the forefront of personal advocacy efforts to change systems. These efforts created the need for a clearer understanding of QOL, including its conceptualization, measurement, and application. This need was met by a group of international QOL practitioners and researchers who developed and published 15 core principles related to QOL's conceptualization, measurement, and application (Schalock et al., 2002). These principles, as revised recently (Schalock, 2005), are summarized in Table 1.1. Note throughout these 12 principles the pervasive themes of equity, inclusion, empowerment, positive growth opportunities, and evidence-based application.

The Current Decade

Research and evaluation efforts during the current decade (2000–2005) have been based largely on the 12 principles summarized in Table 1.1 and have attempted to provide a firmer conceptual and empirical basis for the measurement and application of the QOL construct. Based on this work, a consensus is emerging regarding four guidelines for using QOL-related outcomes (i.e., personal outcomes) for multiple purposes, including personal development, personal well-being, and quality

---

TABLE 1.1

Quality of Life Conceptualization, Measurement, and Application Principles

---

Conceptualization:

1. Quality of life is multidimensional and influenced by personal and environmental factors and their interaction.

2. Quality of life has the same components for all people.

3. Quality of life has both subjective and objective components.

4. Quality of life is enhanced by self-determination, resources, purpose in life, and a sense of belonging.

Measurement:

1. Measurement in quality of life involves the degree to which people have life experiences that they value.

2. Measurement in quality of life reflects the domains that contribute to a full and interconnected life.

3. Measurement in quality of life considers the contexts of physical, social, and cultural environments that are important to people.

4. Measurement in quality of life includes measures of experiences both common to all humans and those unique to individuals.

Application:

1. Quality of life application enhances well-being within cultural contexts.

2. Quality of life principles should be the basis for interventions and supports.

3. Quality of life applications should be evidence based.

4. Quality of life principles should take a prominent place in professional education and training.

---

improvement. These four guidelines are listed in Table 1.2 and discussed more fully below and on subsequent pages.

Recognize the Multidimensionality of Quality of Life

Although chapter 2 expands significantly on this guideline, it is important at this point to state that a life of quality is composed of multiple domains. This notion is shown in Figure 1.1. QOL domains are *the factors composing personal well-being. The set of factors represents the range over which the QOL concept extends and thus defines quality of life.*

Based on a thorough review of the international QOL literature (see Table 2.1),

---

TABLE 1.2

Guidelines for Using Personal Outcomes for Personal Development, Personal Well-Being, and Quality Improvement

---

1. Recognize the multidimensionality of quality of life.

2. Develop indicators for the respective quality of life domains.

3. Assess both subjective and objective quality aspects of quality of life.

4. Focus on the predictors of quality outcomes.

---

most individual-referenced QOL domains fall into one of eight categories: interpersonal relations, social inclusion, personal development, physical well-being, self-determination, material well-being, emotional well-being, and rights. Although the specific listing of domains varies somewhat across investigators (see chapter 2), most suggest that the *number* of domains is less important than the recognition that (a) any proposed QOL model must recognize the need to employ a multi-element framework, (b) individuals know what is important to them, and (c) any set of domains must represent in aggregate the complete QOL construct (Schalock, 2005). It is also important to understand that (a) the relative importance of the above-mentioned eight domains varies among individuals and across one's life span, and (b) although the domains' use differs across respondent and geographical groups, there is good cross-cultural agreement on their importance and factor structure (Jenaro et al., 2005; Schalock et al., 2005).

Develop Quality Indicators
As shown in Figure 1.1, QOL domains are operationalized through quality indicators that are defined as *QOL-related perceptions, behaviors, and conditions that give an indication of a person's well-being.* The personal assessment of one's status on—or aspirations regarding—these indicators are typically reflected in personal outcomes.

Table 1.3 summarizes the most frequently referenced (based on a review of the international QOL literature; Schalock & Verdugo, 2002) quality indicators associated with each of the eight core QOL domains listed earlier. The QOL literature consistently suggests the need to develop specific quality indicators for each QOL domain and to use best-practice measurement methodology for their assessment. This guideline provides a firm conceptual and empirical basis for the measurement and application of the QOL concept and personal outcomes. Once these quality domains and indicators are delineated, they can be assessed by using either subjective (e.g., personal preferences and satisfaction) or objective (e.g., personal experiences and circumstances) methods, such as those described next and in more detail in chapter 3.

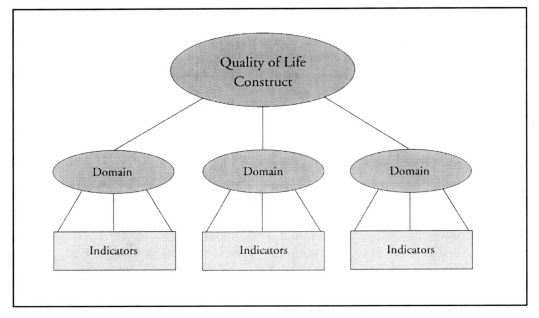

Figure 1.1. Operationalizing the quality of life construct: Domains and indicators.

Assess Subjective and Objective Aspects

One's quality of life has both subjective and objective components. Thus QOL assessment includes the measurement of both subjective well-being (including preferences) and objective life circumstances and experiences. The relationship or correlation between the subjective and objective components is typically quite low (Cummins & Lau, 2004; Perry & Felce 2005a; Schalock & Felce, 2004).

Historically satisfaction has been used to address the subjective nature of quality of life, typically asking individuals how satisfied they are with the various aspects of their lives. The advantages of using satisfaction as a dependent measure in QOL research and evaluation is that it (a) is a commonly used measure of individual life domains (e.g., work, leisure, health), (b) provides an extensive body of research on levels of satisfaction across populations and service delivery recipients, and (c) allows one to assess the relative importance of individual QOL domains and thereby assign value to respective domains. Its major disadvantages are that it (a) demonstrates a trait-like stability over time and correlates little with objective behavioral measures, (b) is sensitive to the tendency toward social desirability and thus may tend to inflate scores (Finlay & Lyons, 2002), (c) is not predicted by environmental conditions, and (d) consistently produces scores around the 70 to 80% level (Cummins, 1998).

On the other hand, the assessment of objective life circumstances and experiences results in better predictors of outcomes related to choice, constructive activities, and social and community well-being (Perry & Felce, 2005b; Schalock & Felce, 2004).

TABLE 1.3
Quality of Life Domains and Quality Indicators

Domain	Most Common Indicators
Emotional well-being	Contentment, self-concept, freedom from stress
Interpersonal relations	Interactions, relationships, supports
Material well-being	Financial status, employment, housing
Personal development	Education, personal competence, performance
Physical well-being	Health care, health status, activities of daily living, recreation or leisure
Self-determination	Autonomy or personal control, goals and personal values, choices
Social inclusion	Community integration and participation, community roles, social support
Rights	Legal and human (dignity and respect)

Note. Summarized from *Handbook on Quality of Life for Human Service Practitioners* (pp. 184–187), by R. L. Schalock and M. A. Verdugo, 2002, Washington, DC: American Association on Mental Retardation.

Thus the following two guidelines are based on the suggestion to assess both subjective and objective quality components (Schalock & Felce, 2004):

1. If one wants to determine whether people with ID-DD are as satisfied with life as other population subgroups, one should assess their level of satisfaction and compare. If the scores are the same, satisfaction is normative. If not, one needs to look for personal or environmental factors that might explain such a difference. However, the expectation that subjective well-being (as measured by levels of satisfaction) will be a sensitive indicator of good environmental design and service programs has yet to be demonstrated.

2. If one wants to evaluate environmental design or service programs for the purposes of performance enhancement or program change, one should use objective indicators of life experiences and circumstances. Examples include physical functioning, stable and predictable environments, social networks and interpersonal relations, community integration and participation, personal competence, employment and living environments, autonomy and personal control, and human and legal rights.

Focus on Predictors of Personal Outcomes
Two significant developments during the current decade related to our understanding of personal outcomes and their use have been (a) the development of program logic

models (Andrews, 2004; Kaplan & Garrett, 2005; Schalock & Bonham, 2003), and (b) the use of multivariate research designs (Gardner & Carran, 2005; Perry & Felce, 2005b; Schalock, 2004).

Program logic models make a distinction among *program inputs* (i.e., resources), *program processes* (e.g., individualized services and supports), *program outputs* (e.g., number of program participants and time spent in the program), and *program outcomes* (e.g., personal outcomes, quality indicators, performance indicators). This distinction has focused our attention on personal outcomes and factors that predict these outcomes (Schalock & Bonham, 2003).

Multivariate research designs are used to determine the significant predictors of personal outcomes. The design is very different from a "between groups" design that focuses on comparing individuals' scores. Although comparisons are sometimes used at the individual and organizational level, the current emphasis is on understanding the significant predictors of personal outcomes and then using this information for quality improvement (Schalock & Bonham, 2003; Schalock, Bonham, & Marchand, 2000). Across a number of studies (e.g., Perry & Felce, 2005b; Schalock & Verdugo, 2002), the following personal characteristics, environmental variables, and provider characteristics significantly predict QOL outcomes:

- Personal characteristics: health status and adaptive behavior level

- Environmental variables: perceived social supports, type of residential setting, number of household activities participated in, transportation availability, earnings, and integrated activities

- Provider characteristics: work stress score, satisfaction working with client, staff attention, and job satisfaction

The implication of these significant predictors for personal outcomes is obvious: Organizations and systems need to focus on what they can do to (a) enhance health status and adaptive behavior; (b) provide or facilitate social supports, more independent and productive environments, and community involvement; and (c) maximize working conditions that result in increased staff job satisfaction and reduced employee stress. Consistent with these suggestions is the significant work done during the latter part of the previous decade regarding the significant factors that effect quality improvement. Chief among these factors are (a) the importance of stakeholder involvement in planning and evaluation, (b) the use of evaluation information for programmatic change or improvement, (c) the key roles that both the program's internal and external environments play in the use of results and programmatic change, (d) the need to influence decision makers' understanding of—and commitment to—change based on evaluation data, (e) the necessity of changing people's behavior to focus on the predictors of personal outcomes and what they can do to influence those predictors, and (f) the realistic potential for individuals and organizations to learn and change

(Hodges & Hernandez, 1999; Schalock & Bonham, 2003).

In summary, the four guidelines just discussed and listed in Table 1.2 are critical to both the measurement of personal quality outcomes as discussed in chapter 3, and the implementation of quality improvement as discussed in part 4. These guidelines also reflect the differences between personal outcomes and social indicators. This distinction is briefly discussed next.

Social Indicators Versus Personal Outcomes

Social Indicators

Social indicators generally refer to external, environmentally based conditions such as health, social welfare, friendships, standard of living, education, public safety, employment rates, literacy, mortality, life expectancy, housing, neighborhood, and leisure. These indicators may be defined as a statistic of direct normative interest that facilitates concise, comprehensive, and balanced judgments about the conditions of major aspects of society (Andrews & Whithey, 1976). Such indicators are good for measuring the collective quality of community or national life; however, they are insufficient to measure an individual's perceived personal well-being or quality outcomes from rehabilitation programs. Campbell, Converse, and Rogers (1976) argue, for example, that social indicators reflect only an outsider's judgment of quality as suggested by external, environmentally based conditions.

Personal Outcomes

In distinction, personal outcomes focus on the individual and those factors that contribute to one's personal well-being. As used throughout the text, personal outcomes are person-defined and valued QOL aspirations. Thus, while social indicators describe the life quality of particular national subgroups and compare them with more general national populations, personal outcomes are generally defined within the context of QOL domains and indicators. They reflect the increased concern for the social and psychological dynamics of perceived well-being, including factors related to social support and integration, internal control, autonomy or independence, self-confidence, aspirations and expectations, and values having to do with family, job, and life in general (Deci, 2004; Turnbull, Brown, & Turnbull, 2004).

There is another major difference between social indicators and personal outcomes; this relates to the notion of normative interest. Although that interest is key to the use and understanding of social indicators, current best practices in the area of personal outcomes minimize the use of normative and comparative judgments. The individual *is* the point of reference in personal outcomes, and any comparison should be *within* the person and not between individuals.

This difference is very important to understand from two perspectives. First, at its core the QOL concept provides (a) a sense of reference and guidance from the individual's perspective, (b) an overriding principle to enhance an individual's well-being and collaborate for change at the organizational and systems level, and (c) a common language and systematic framework to guide quality improvement. Second, personal outcomes reflect the increased interest in how time-related phenomena link to life quality and the relative importance of the respective QOL domains across the life span.

Personal Outcomes and Evaluation Theory

Program evaluation theory and strategies have changed in three significant ways over the past two decades (Schalock, 2001). This volume's approach to the assessment and use of personal outcomes reflects these three changes.

First, a theory-driven approach to program evaluation has emerged that explains how program inputs (e.g., a QOL focus and emphasis) and external factors influence personal outcomes. In addition to helping one understand how programs work, a theory-driven approach identifies and prioritizes evaluation questions and aligns evaluation methodology to answering those questions (Chen, 1990; Donaldson & Gooler, 2003).

Second, methodological pluralism, which combines qualitative and quantitative data-gathering strategies and recognizes the key role played by all stakeholders, has emerged as the principal method for assessing quality indicators or personal outcomes (Denzin & Lincoln, 2000; Fishman, 2003; Schalock, 2005).

Third, utilization-focused evaluation has become the norm. This approach emphasizes that (a) evaluation should not focus solely on outcomes, but also on the structure and causal entities that produce the outcomes; (b) learning organizations can use evaluation information for programmatic change and improved personal outcomes; and (c) information should be used to modify or change the structures or causal entities (Hodges & Hernandez, 1999; House, 1991; Newcomer, 1997; Patton, 1997).

Summary

In summary, the QOL construct provides the framework for personal outcomes and quality improvement. As currently used the QOL concept is important as (a) a sensitizing notion that gives us a sense of reference and guidance from the individual's perspective focusing on the person and the individual's environment, (b) a conceptual framework for assessing quality indicators or personal outcomes, (c) a social construct that guides performance enhancement strategies, and (d) a criterion for assessing the effectiveness of those strategies.

The QOL concept has evolved from a sensitizing notion to a change agent. As the concept has evolved, policies and practices related to people with ID-DD have also changed. These changes will be evident in subsequent chapters that discuss the measurement and use of quality indicators or personal outcomes at the organizational and systems level.

As the QOL concept has evolved, our research methodology has also changed. The emphasis now is on making use of quality domains and indicators, and using both quantitative and qualitative methods to identify predictor and outcome variables. In that regard, throughout the chapter we've noted the critical importance of (a) understanding and implementing core conceptualization, measurement, and application principles (Table 1.1); (b) employing key guidelines for using personal outcomes for personal development, personal well-being, and quality improvement (Table 1.2); and (c) distinguishing between personal outcomes and social indicators. These processes allow one to align one's QOL model with quality indicators and measured personal outcomes.

At its core, the QOL concept makes us think differently about service recipients and the personal outcomes they experience. Although today we understand much better the factors that comprise a life of quality from the individual's perspective, there is a need for the reader to appreciate the significant work that has been done to clarify quality domains and indicators. That work is summarized in the following chapter.

CHAPTER 2

Quality Domains and Indicators

Introduction and Overview

In chapter 1 we discussed the logical progression from a *quality of life (QOL) model*, to *quality domains*, to *quality indicators* whose measurement results in *personal outcomes*. This chapter focuses primarily on quality indicators that are defined as *QOL-related perceptions, behaviors, and conditions that give an indication of a person's well-being*.

Before reviewing the currently published QOL domains and indicators, we note two points. First, the focus of the text is primarily on person-centered QOL domains and indicators, even though considerable work is currently being done on family quality of life. (The interested reader is referred to the work of Poston et al. [2003] and Summers et al. [2005] for a detailed description of that work.) Second, it is important to understand the context and use of core indicators and the key role they play in establishing personal outcomes for individuals with intellectual disabilities and developmental disabilities (ID-DD). This discussion is presented on subsequent pages. Thereafter the chapter (a) summarizes the numerous quality domains and indicators that are currently available, and (b) discusses 10 criteria to use when selecting a set of quality indicators to serve as the basis for measuring of personal outcomes.

Quality Indicators: Context and Use

Context

The concept of quality indicators has emerged over the past three decades in conjunction with the QOL concept and our attempts to conceptualize, measure, and apply it to people with ID-DD. As discussed in chapter 1, during the 1980s the field first embraced the QOL concept, but not until the 1990s and the current decade did a consensus emerge regarding its multidimensionality and the need to develop measurable indicators of personal outcomes.

TABLE 2.1

Changing Approaches to Accountability

Era	Focus	Outcomes
Institutional reforms	Protection, health, safety	Quality assurance; accreditation
Deinstitutionalization	Habilitation planning	IHP; accreditation
Community options	Independence, productivity, community integration	IPP; personal outcomes
Supports model	Empowerment, inclusion, person-centered planning, quality of life	ISP; personal well-being, quality outcomes

Note. IHP = individual habilitation plan. IPP = individual program plan. ISP = individual supports plan.

The context of quality indicators can also be viewed from an accountability perspective that relates desired outcomes to service provision eras and respective delivery foci. Table 2.1, for example, shows how program focus and desired accountability outcomes have changed in the field during recent eras of institutional reform, deinstitutionalization, community options, and the supports paradigm (Gardner & Nudler, 1999).

Useful Purposes

Quality indicators provide the conceptual and empirical link between the quality revolution, with its focus on valued, person-referenced outcomes, and the reform movement, with its emphasis on outputs rather than inputs and quality improvement (Chelimsky & Shadish, 1995; Schalock, 2001). As such, they are useful for at least five purposes, summarized in Table 2.2 and discussed below.

Allow Measurement of Multiple Dimensions

First, quality indicators allow one to put into measurable form (i.e., operationalize) the multiple dimensions of quality of life. For example, the QOL domain of self-determination may not be easily understood until it is defined and measured on the basis of the individual establishing personal goals, making personal choices, and exerting

---

TABLE 2.2
Five Useful Purposes of Quality Indicators

---

1. Allow measurement of the multiple dimensions of quality of life.

2. Facilitate accountability through the measurement of personal outcomes.

3. Permit reporting, program enhancement, and advocating for change at the level of the individual, organization, system, and community.

4. Provide a framework for best practices regarding discovery, remediation, and quality improvement.

5. Demonstrate stability across groups and sensitivity to people's perceptions.

---

autonomy and personal control. Similarly, emotional well-being may be an elusive QOL domain until it is defined and measured in regard to the individual's perceived degree of contentment, demonstrated self-concept, and observed freedom from stress. This use of quality indicators allows users to (a) increase communication among important stakeholders, (b) measure the factors or domains comprising personal well-being, and (c) recognize the multidimensionality and the holistic perspective of the QOL concept.

Facilitate Accountability
Second, quality indicators allow one to meet the increasing need to be accountable in terms of personal outcomes. For example, the state of Nebraska Division of Developmental Disabilities annually publishes information on Nebraska's developmental disabilities service providers and the assessed quality of life of individuals receiving those services (Ferdinand & Smith, 2002; Keith & Bonham, 2005). Among other things, each service provider is profiled in regard to his or her clientele's average QOL scores (along with scores for individuals without disabilities living in the same communities) for the following quality indicators: satisfaction, competence/productivity, empowerment/independence, social belonging/community integration, rights, relationships, economic security, growth and development, and perception of well-being. This use of quality indicators or outcomes represents one state's accountability efforts; it also shows how personal outcomes can be used for appraisal purposes, focusing on an individual or an organization.

Permit Reporting, Program Enhancement, and Advocacy
Third, quality indicators lend themselves to multiple uses, including reporting (e.g., as just described for Nebraska), quality improvement (as described in chap. 3 regarding the state of Maryland Ask Me! Project), and organizational and systems change. Throughout the world such change is reflected in (a) individuals advocating for

increased self-advocacy, self-determination, empowerment, and personal development opportunities; (b) organizations and systems using measured quality indicators for improvement that emphasizes dimensions of quality services, such as reliability, responsiveness, empathy, extensiveness, and appropriateness; (c) quality improvement techniques being implemented based on QOL domains, personal outcomes, quality indicators, and significant predictors of personal outcomes; and (d) the incorporation of key QOL concepts and principles into public policy (Schalock, 2005; Schalock & Verdugo, 2002).

Provide a Framework for Best Practices

Fourth, quality indicators provide a framework for best practices. For example, the Centers for Medicare and Medicaid Home and Community-Based Services' Quality Framework model (discussed in chap. 6) supports efforts to provide desired person-referenced outcomes across seven dimensions: participant access, participant-centered service planning and delivery, provider capacity and capabilities, participant safeguards, participant rights and responsibilities, participant outcomes and satisfaction, and system performance. These outcomes are enhanced through program design and management with three critical goals: (a) discovery: collecting data and information about direct participant experiences in order to assess the program's ongoing implementation, identifying strengths and opportunities for improvement; (b) remediation: taking action to remedy specific problems or concerns; and (c) continuous quality improvement that involves using data and quality-related information to effect improved program operations.

Demonstrate Stability and Sensitivity

Fifth, quality indicators are sensitive to respondent and geographical group differences and can thereby demonstrate both stability across groups and sensitivity to people's perceptions. For example, a recently published cross-cultural study (Schalock et al., 2005) involved surveying three respondent groups (individuals with disabilities, parents, and professionals; N = 2,500) representing five geographical groups (Spain, Central and South America, Canada, mainland China, and the United States) on the importance and use of the 24 quality indicators listed in Table 1.3. Results indicated that (a) there were similar profiles on importance and use across the respondent and geographical groups, but groups differed on the frequency per response category; (b) there were significant differences in mean QOL importance and use scores for both the respondent and geographical groupings; and (c) factors on importance and use generally grouped into the eight QOL domains listed in Table 1.3. The importance of this study is that it demonstrates both the *stability* of measured quality indicators across groups and the *sensitivity* of the indicators to differences in individual perceptions. As discussed later in this chapter, these two characteristics are essential criteria in the selection and use of quality indicators as the basis for measuring personal outcomes.

In summary, quality indicators have emerged within the context of the quality revolution and the reform movement. As summarized in Table 2.2, their importance and use relate to measurement, reporting, quality improvement, and advocating for change at the individual, organizational, systems, and wider community levels. Because of their stability across groups and their sensitivity to individual differences, they provide a framework for best practices. Examples of these uses are elaborated in parts 2 and 3 of the text. In the meantime, we need to review the currently reported quality indicators and their respective quality domains.

Quality Domains and Quality Indicators

Due to the ubiquity of QOL definitions, models, and domains, it is necessary to synthesize this vast amount of information into a workable model for implementing personal outcomes. In this section of the chapter, we do two things. First, we present results of a content analysis of recent literature in the field of ID-DD as related to individual-referenced QOL domains. This analysis identifies clearly the life experiences and circumstances reflective of quality indicators and potential personal outcomes. Second, we present those QOL domains and indicators with which we three authors have been working at the individual, organizational, and systems levels. These three listings are based on considerable development and validation work and have a list of associated empirically derived quality indicators. In addition to these domains and indicators, we summarize other commonly referenced investigators and their respective QOL domains and indicators. Thus, by the end of this chapter section, readers should have a good appreciation and understanding of optional quality domains and associated quality indicators, allowing them to consider which domains and measured indicators are potentially valuable and useful to them. The final section of the chapter presents criteria for selecting a set of quality indicators to use as the basis for the measurement of personal outcomes.

Content Analysis of Individual-Referenced QOL Factors

Sixteen sources (research articles, book chapters, or books) regarding individual-referenced QOL domains were analyzed to determine the factors included in respective QOL models. A listing was made of the factors found, along with a tabulation of the frequency of each factor reported across the 16 sources. The results of this analysis are presented in Table 2.3. The following factors are most commonly referenced in the ID-DD QOL literature: interpersonal relations, social inclusion, personal development, physical well-being, self-determination, material well-being, emotional well-being, and rights. The next tier is composed of factors related to living environment, family, recreation and leisure, and safety and security. As discussed in the following section, these factors are reflected in the QOL models and respective QOL domains and indicators used by the authors.

Quality Domains and Associated Quality Indicators

Considerable conceptual and empirical work underlies three sets of QOL-related domains and their respective indicators. These are QOL domains, summarized in Table 2.4 (Schalock & Verdugo, 2002), personal outcomes, summarized in Table 2.5 (Council on Quality and Leadership, 1997, 2000d; Gardner & Carran, 2005; Gardner & Nudler, 1999), and core domains, summarized in Table 2.6 (Human Services

TABLE 2.3	
Quality Factors: Content Analysis of Individual-Referenced Domains	
Factor	**Times Referenced (out of 16 articles)**
Interpersonal relations	16
Social inclusion	15
Personal development	14
Physical well-being	13
Self-determination	13
Material well-being	13
Emotional well-being	9
Rights	8
Environment (home, residence, living situation)	6
Family	5
Recreation and leisure	5
Safety or security	4
Satisfaction	3

Note. Based on individual-referenced QOL domains published by Bonham et al. (2004), Cummins (1997a, 1997b, 2003), Felce & Perry (1996), Ferdinand & Smith (2002), Gardner & Nudler (1997), Gettings & Bradley (1997), Harner & Heal (1993), Hughes et al. (1995), Karon & Bernard (2002), Karon, Stegemann, & Barnard (2003), Renwick, Brown, & Raphael (2000), Schalock & Keith (1993), Schalock & Verdugo (2002), World Health Organization QOL Group (1995).

Research Institute & National Association of State Directors of Developmental Disabilities Services, 2003). In addition, Table 2.7 lists the quality domains and indicators proposed by commonly referenced QOL investigators who are not included in Tables 2.4–2.6.

TABLE 2.4	
Quality of Life Domains and Associated Quality Indicators	
Domain	**Indicators and Descriptors**
Emotional well-being	Contentment (satisfaction, moods, enjoyment) Self-concept (identity, self-worth, self-esteem) Lack of stress (predictability and control)
Interpersonal relations	Interactions (social networks, social contacts) Relationships (family, friends, peers) Supports (emotional, physical, financial, feedback)
Material well-being	Financial status (income, benefits) Employment (work status, work environment) Housing (type of residence, ownership)
Personal development	Education (achievements, status) Personal competence (cognitive, social, practical) Performance (success, achievement, productivity)
Physical well-being	Health (functioning, symptoms, fitness, nutrition) Activities of daily living (self-care skills, mobility) Leisure (recreation, hobbies)
Self-determination	Autonomy or personal control (independence) Goals and personal values (desires, expectations) Choices (opportunities, options, preferences)
Social inclusion	Community integration and participation Community roles (contributor, volunteer) Social supports (support network, services)
Rights	Human (respect, dignity, equality) Legal (citizenship, access, due process)

Note. Summarized from *Handbook on Quality of Life for Human Service Practitioners* (pp. 184–187), by R. L. Schalock and M. A. Verdugo, 2002, Washington, DC: American Association on Mental Retardation.

TABLE 2.5 Personal Outcome Measures and Associated Quality Indicators	
Domain	**Indicators**
Identity	People choose personal goals. People choose where and with whom to live. People choose where they work. People have intimate relationships. People are satisfied with services. People are satisfied with their personal life situations.
Autonomy	People choose their daily routines. People have time, space, and opportunity for privacy. People decide when to share personal information. People use their environments.
Affiliation	People live in integrated environments. People participate in the life of the community. People interact with other members of the community. People perform different social roles. People have friends. People are respected.
Attainment	People choose services. People realize personal goals.
Safeguards	People remain connected to natural supports. People are safe.
Rights	People exercise rights. People are treated fairly.
Health and wellness	People have the best possible health. People are free from abuse and neglect. People experience continuity and security.

Note. From *Personal Outcome Measures*, by the Council on Quality and Leadership, 1997, 2000. Towson, MD. Reprinted with permission.

TABLE 2.6 **Core Domains and Associated Quality Indicators**	
Domain	**Concerns and Indicators**
Work	**Concern:** *People have support to find and maintain community integrated employment.* **Indicators:** The average monthly earnings of people who have community jobs The percentage of people earning at or above the state minimum wage The average number of hours worked per month in these jobs Of people who have a job in the community, the percentage who were continuously employed during the previous year Of people who have a job in the community, the percentage who receive job benefits Of people who have a job in the community, the average length of time people have been working at their current jobs The proportion of all individuals who receive daytime supports for any type who are engaged in community integrated employment
Community inclusion	**Concern:** *People have support to participate in everyday community activities.* **Indicator:** The proportion of people who participate in everyday integrated activities in their communities
Choices and decisions	**Concern:** *People make choices about their lives and are actively engaged in planning their services and supports.* **Indicators:** The proportion of people who make choices about their everyday lives, including housing, roommates, daily routines, jobs, support staff or providers, and social activities

(table continues)

TABLE 2.6 *(continued)*	
Domain	**Concerns and Indicators**
Self-determination	**Concern:** *People have authority and are supported to direct and manage their own services.* **Indicator:** The proportion of people who control their own budgets
Relationships	**Concern:** *People have friends and relationships.* **Indicators:** The proportion of people who have friends and caring relationships with people other than support staff and family members The proportion of people who have a close friend, someone they can talk to about personal feelings The proportion of people who are able to see their families and friends when they want The proportion of people who feel lonely
Satisfaction	**Concern:** *People are satisfied with the services and supports they receive.* **Indicators:** The proportion of people who are satisfied with where they live The proportion of people who are satisfied with their jobs or day programs The proportion of people who are satisfied with [life in general, personal life]

Note. Adapted from *National Core Indicators: 5 Years of Performance Measurement*, by Human Services Research Institute and National Association of State Directors of Developmental Disabilities Services (HSRI & NASDDDS), 2003. Cambridge, MA, & Alexandria, VA. Reprinted with permission.

Note. The six domains listed above are for the larger domain of consumer outcomes. Other domains included in the National Core Indicators are systems performance; health, welfare, and rights; staff stability and competence; family indicators; and case management.

Two significant patterns emerge from an analysis of the quality indicators listed in Tables 2.4–2.7. First, the vast majority use person-referenced indicators, with a few extending beyond the person to the family and person-centered services. Second,

	TABLE 2.7 Commonly Referenced Investigators and Respective Quality Domains and Indicators	
Investigator	**Quality Domains and Indicators**
Cummins (1997a)	Material well-being, health, productivity, intimacy, safety, place in community, emotional well-being
Felce & Perry (1996)	Physical well-being, material well-being, social well-being, development and activity, emotional well-being
Hughes et al. (1995)	Social relations and interactions, psychological well-being and personal satisfaction, employment, self-determination, autonomy and personal choice, recreation and leisure, personal competence, community adjustment and independent living skills, community integration, normalization, personal development and fulfillment, social acceptance, social status and ecological fit, physical and material well-being, civic responsibility
Renwick, Brown, & Raphael (2000)	Physical well-being, psychological being, spiritual being, physical belonging, social belonging community belonging, practical becoming, leisure becoming, growth becoming
World Health Organization QOL Group (1995)	Physical, psychological, level of independence, social relationships, environment, spiritual/personal beliefs

there is considerable agreement across the quality indicators as well as the QOL domains basic to the indicators. These two patterns are good news in that they validate the results of the content analysis presented in Table 2.3 and indicate a general consensus among QOL investigators. Thus there is no reason to recommend one list over another, but to familiarize the reader with a number of criteria that should be used in selecting quality indicators to measure and use as the basis for quality outcomes. These criteria are discussed in the next section.

Criteria for Selecting Quality Indicators

Potential users need to be sensitive to a number of general considerations when selecting specific quality indicators. In this regard, we authors are aware of the delicate balance between measurement of personal quality of life and measurement of program performance. We are also aware that we are slowly making the transition from quality indicators that are program driven to indicators that are personally defined and driven by personal goals and aspirations. Thus those criteria for selecting quality indicators listed in Table 2.8 reflect the concern of program managers but also recognize that people are as important as programs.

The following six considerations reflect our "transitional" status. First, the indicators should reflect what people want in their lives. Second, the indicators selected need to reflect the sphere of a program or system's influence and activity and thus encompass desired goals and personal outcomes. Third, one needs to select quality indicators that are aligned with their intended use. For example, the criteria listed in Table 2.8 for selecting quality indicators that focus only on the individual are less extensive than those focusing on the organization or system. Similarly, if the purpose of the quality indicators is primarily personal appraisal, the selection criteria are less extensive than if they are to be used for organization-level quality improvement, systems-level policy analysis, or research. Fourth, selected quality indicators need to be meaningful and interpreted by a homogeneous constituency. Although stakeholders vary across organizations and systems, the need for clear communication and consistent terminology is sought by all stakeholders, whether they are service recipients, family members, program staff, administrators, policy makers, funders, or society at large. Fifth, selected quality indicators and their measurement need to be within the organization or system's data collection and analysis capability; data collection and analysis take time, money, and expertise. Sixth, the individual, organization, or system needs to be committed to monitor the selected quality indicators over time. Quality indicators and personal outcomes change due to individual choice, developmental milestones, and/or the services and supports people receive. Thus the selection of quality indicators needs to be thought of as a dynamic, not a static, process.

With these general considerations in mind, 10 criteria for selecting quality indicators are presented in Table 2.8. Although on the surface these 10 criteria appear straightforward (and indeed they are), potential users need to address some important considerations.

1. One's QOL model must be aligned to respective quality domains and indicators, and indicators must be sensitive to change and reflect personal well-being. This consideration underscores the importance of maintaining fidelity to one's overall conceptual model for approaching quality domains, indicators, and personal outcomes.

2. Individuals value many things, some of which may not fit into a list of quality indicators.

TABLE 2.8
Criteria for Selecting Quality Indicators

The quality indicators selected should:

1. Have face validity with those people involved (i.e., individuals and families).

2. Be measurable and psychometrically sound.

3. Be conceptually related to a quality of life (QOL) model and reflect the range over which the QOL concept extends (and thus defines quality of life).

4. Have potential for improvement that maximizes personal well-being.

5. Be easily understood and readily communicated (simplicity).

6. Be those that the provider has some direct or indirect control over.

7. Be considered as a template by which organizations, systems, and states can judge current status and base future efforts.

8. Reflect innovation, robustness, and cost-efficiency.

9. Be comprehensive.

10. Reflect phenomena that are neither too rare nor too common. If too rare, they will not occur frequently enough to identify trends and reasonable benchmarks; if too common, they may not show sufficient change or fluctuation.

---

3. In regard to quality indicators or personal outcomes, a typical assumption is made: that services and supports are clearly defined, are largely under the control of the service provider, and have an impact on the service recipient. Although this is a valid assumption, one needs to be aware of this consideration and be selective in one's choice of quality indicators. In that deliberation, Schalock (1997) suggests you think about some of the fears that various constituents have about quality indicators and quality outcomes due to (a) the distortion of programs to meet the expected results, (b) the responsibility for both progress and failure that cannot be accurately described, and (c) the fact that true causes of personal change are often outside the control of those held accountable.

4. Although the QOL concept is increasingly used as an agent for organizational and quality improvement rather than for comparison purposes, one still finds such comparative uses in evaluative research, policy analysis, and systems analysis. Anyone using quality indicators and personal outcomes for such purposes needs to understand fully the measurement and methodological issues discussed in chapter 3.

5. One needs to be sensitive to what some program evaluators (e.g., Schalock, 2001;

Wholey 1987) refer to as an organization's or system's "evaluability" and the degree to which it is feasible for the entity (i.e., organization or system) to assess and use quality indicators and personal outcomes. In terms of evaluability, one must consider three organizational and systems characteristics when selecting the type and number of quality indicators to be assessed and used for reporting and quality enhancement: (a) the entity's *attitude* and commitment to information (i.e., data) and its use; (b) the presence of evaluation *catalysts,* such as internal motivation (e.g., self-advocates) or external (e.g., accreditation or certification); and (c) the presence (or absence) of the necessary *ingredients,* including data sets, a data management system, and expertise (i.e., time, money, and skills). These three factors—attitude, catalysts, and ingredients—need to be considered in the selection and use of quality indicators.

Numerous models have been developed to improve information use. Common themes (as discussed more fully in parts 2–4) among these models include: (a) the importance of stakeholder involvement in planning and implementation, (b) the use of information for quality improvement, (c) the key roles played by the program's internal and external environments in the use of results, (d) the need to influence decision makers' understanding of—and commitment to—change based on the quality outcomes, (e) the necessity of changing leadership styles, and (f) the realistic potential for organizational learning (Johnson, 1998; Patton, 1997).

Summary

Quality domains and indicators are the bridge between a QOL model and measured personal outcomes. Thus their conceptualization and selection are essential components in determining personal outcomes for people with ID-DD and implementing quality improvement. The purpose of this chapter has been to describe the context, use, and importance of quality indicators, and to review and summarize the currently published quality indicators and the QOL models and quality domains on which they are based. We also considered 10 criteria for selecting quality indicators, defined as QOL-related perceptions, behaviors, or conditions that give an indication of the person's well-being.

Those interested in using quality indicators should first (a) understand their importance and use (Table 2.2), (b) appreciate the extensive literature regarding quality factors (Tables 2.3), (c) be familiar with published QOL-related domains and indicators (Tables 2.4–2.7), and (d) be familiar with potential criteria for selecting quality indicators (Table 2.8). This foundational understanding provides the basis for approaching the measurement of quality indicators and personal outcomes—the topic of chapter 3.

Measuring Personal Outcomes: An Information Collection Process

Introduction and Overview

Measuring personal outcomes involves more than instruments and psychometrics. It is a process that begins with the individual as *the* key informant and ends with quality improvement and its effects. Thus measuring personal outcomes requires one to think differently about traditional measurement procedures and practices. Although not replacing the need to demonstrate reliable and valid measurement strategies, measuring personal outcomes requires a *broad information collection process*. That process provides the framework for this chapter.

In the previous chapter, we discussed the context and use of quality indicators that were defined as quality of life (QOL)-related perceptions, behaviors, and conditions that give an indication of a person's well-being. We also summarized the currently published QOL domains and their respective indicators (Tables 2.4–2.7) and suggested 10 criteria (Table 2.8) to use when selecting a set of quality indicators to serve as the basis for measuring personal outcomes.

The purpose of this chapter is to discuss an information collection process that results in personal outcomes that can be used for a number of purposes, including quality improvement. As you read the chapter, keep in mind that although personal outcomes can be used at the organizational or systems level, their assessment is made at the individual level and based primarily on an in-person interview.

The chapter begins with a general discussion of the value of measuring outcomes and gives four measurement principles that guide the process. Thereafter the chapter (a) discusses the characteristics of an information collection process and suggests guidelines and ethical principles necessary to its successful implementation, and (b) summarizes four key procedural issues basic to measuring personal outcomes (i.e., interviewing techniques, the use of proxies, meeting psychometric standards, and overcoming methodological issues related to aggregating individual-referenced data at the organizational and systems level). The chapter concludes with an example of how the information collection process addresses these four procedural issues and results in personal outcomes that provide the basis for quality improvement.

The Value of Measuring Personal Outcomes

The value of measuring personal outcomes can be viewed from two perspectives: (a) as a focus for our thinking, and (b) as a basis for responsive management.

In this first regard, personal outcomes are important to all people and should be thought of in the same way for all people. Assessing personal outcomes requires (a) an understanding of the degree to which people experience a good life, (b) a valuing of quality within people's lives, and (c) a desire to maintain and enhance the things that can add quality to their lives. Measuring quality should never support maintaining or encouraging a low quality of life for anyone. In addition, any assessment of personal outcomes should be based on the view that all people share the human experience together and that every human being is entitled to live a good life within his or her society. This central belief is the principal ethical criterion to use when measuring personal outcomes.

In regard to responsive management, there is value in measuring personal outcomes. Hakes (2001), for example, suggests the following six benefits: (a) Focusing on outcomes counters a tendency to overemphasize the inputs; (b) such measurement directs more time and attention toward results; (c) it provides a basis for legitimately bragging about accomplishments; (d) it promotes healthy communication among consumers, employees, and managers; (e) it facilitates early identification and correction of problems at the source before they require correcting from the outside; and (f) at the most basic level, the value of measuring personal outcomes is that they tell us what is and is not working.

These values are reflected in measurement principles developed and validated by a group of international QOL investigators (Schalock et al., 2002; Schalock, 2005). These four principles, described more fully in Table 3.1, are that measurement in quality of life: (a) involves the degree to which people have life experiences that they value; (2) reflects the domains that contribute to a full and interconnected life; (c) considers the contexts of physical, social, and cultural environments that are important to people; and (d) includes measures of experiences both common to all humans and unique to individuals.

Measurement as an Information Collection Process

A Two-Component Information Collection Process

The purpose of this chapter section is not to summarize the rich and extensive array of instruments used to assess individual-referenced quality outcomes. (The interested

---

TABLE 3.1

Principles Underlying the Measurement of Quality Outcomes

Principle 1. *Measurement in quality of life involves the degree to which people have life experiences that they value.* This means that measurement:

- focuses on key aspects of life that can be improved;

- is carried out for a clear, practical purpose that supports people moving toward better lives;

- is described within a framework that it potentially positive, neutral, and negative— suggesting that it is possible to move toward the very positive;

- is interpreted within the context of an overall life-span approach.

Principle 2. *Measurement in quality of life reflects the domains that contribute to a full and interconnected life.* This means that

- measurement uses a broad range of life domains;

- quantitative measurement uses key indicators of a life of quality;

- qualitative measurement procedures explore and describe a range of aspects within each domain.

Principle 3. *Measurement in quality of life considers the contexts of physical, social, and cultural environments that are important to people.* This means that

- the measurement framework is based on well-established theory of broad life concepts;

- one recognizes that the meaning of life experiences that are positively valued varies across time and among cultures;

- the measurement framework provides a clear way to demonstrate the positive values of life;

- the measuring of quality outcomes from the perspective of people not able to speak for themselves should use applicable methods such as observation and participant observation;

- proxy measures of subjective well-being (e.g., satisfaction) should be clearly identified as representing another person's perspective;

- interpretation is made within the context of the person's environment.

(table continues)

TABLE 3.1 *(continued)*

Principle 4. *Measurement in quality of life includes measures of experiences both common to all humans and those unique to individuals.* This means that

- measurement uses both subjective and objective indicators;

- measurement uses both qualitative and quantitative measures;

- subjective measures reflect the individual's level of satisfaction and objective measures reflect the individual's personal experiences and circumstances.

---

reader is referred to Cummins, 2003, 2004a, 2004b, who lists more than 600 and/or Schalock & Verdugo, 2002, who list more than 250.) Rather, our purpose is to have the reader think beyond instruments and their psychometric properties to a two-component information collection process for measuring personal outcomes within a QOL context.

The first component involves an in-person interview that identifies those QOL indicators valued by the person (i.e., personal outcomes).

The second is to then place these desired personal outcomes within the context of community indicators and evaluate the discrepancy between the two. As we discuss in chapters 9 and 10, the function of quality improvement is to reduce the discrepancy.

This two-component process integrates the subjective and objective levels of measurement discussed in the previous chapter and emphasizes personally defined outcomes. It is also consistent with person-centered planning, individualized supports, and self-advocacy. Its implementation rests on guidelines and principles, as discussed below.

Information Collection Guidelines
QOL-related information is important, and its measurement needs to be guided by both specific guidelines and ethical principles. Table 3.2 summarizes eight guidelines undergirding the implementation of an information collection process. These guidelines reflect a number of key points discussed throughout the text: (a) the emphasis on personally defined outcomes, (b) the use of objective indicators related to personal experiences and circumstances against which personally defined outcomes can be evaluated, (c) the use of psychometrically sound instruments and procedures, (d) the alignment of personal outcomes with objective conditions within the community, and finally (e) the purpose of measuring personal outcomes is to improve individual quality of life.

Ethical Principles
Individuals involved in the measurement of personal outcomes should be deeply

---

TABLE 3.2

Guidelines for Collecting Quality of Life Information

---

1. Surveys should reflect what individuals value; considering this, the person with ID-DD needs to be present from the beginning.

2. Interviewers need to be competent in the administration of the particular protocol (i.e., survey). Competency can be demonstrated in a variety of ways, including observation, mock interviews, and work samples.

3. The provider assumes responsibility for collecting the data and linking that information to quality improvement.

4. Collecting data and implementing quality improvement strategies should be viewed as a partnership among key stakeholders.

5. Scheduling of the information collection process should be determined by the individual.

6. The purposes of the process are to improve individual quality of life, enhance community life, and improve systems performance.

7. The process should reflect respect for people's rights, dignity, and privacy.

8. Evidence and allegations of abuse, neglect, or exploitation should be reported immediately to a responsible person.

---

concerned about the impact their results may have on the individual and organization (Newman & Brown, 1996). Thus the measurement of personal outcomes needs to be based not only on an information collection process (as just discussed), but also guided by the following ethical principles (Academy of Human Resource Development, 1999; American Evaluation Association, 1995; Beauchamp & Childress, 1983):

- Nonmalficience (i.e., do no harm)

- Fidelity to a QOL model

- Beneficience (i.e., the quality of doing good, taking positive steps to help others, or the notion that one ought to do or promote actions that benefit others)

- Competence (i.e., adherence to technical standards and accurate and detailed reporting)

- Systemic inquiry (i.e., exploring with stakeholders the shortcomings and strengths of the questions asked and the various approaches that might be used to answer questions)

- Respect for people (i.e., maximizing benefits, reducing harm, and identifying and respecting differences)

The measurement of QOL-related personal outcomes not only relies on those guidelines and ethical principles just discussed, but also calls for a thorough understanding of procedural issues.

Measuring Personal Outcomes: Procedural Issues

Four procedural issues must be understood by people measuring QOL-related personal outcomes: interviewing techniques, the use of proxies, meeting psychometric standards, and overcoming issues related to the aggregation of individual data to the organizational or systems level.

Interviewing Techniques

When measuring personal outcomes, the individual is the primary data source. Thus interviewers need to be both competent in interviewing techniques and sensitive to factors associated with the interviewee. Tassé, Schalock, Thompson, and Wehmeyer (2005) discuss the following issues an interviewer must consider: (a) recognizing that disability is often associated with stigma; people with ID-DD do not want to be viewed as incapable, incompetent, or devalued; (b) realizing that at times people with ID-DD want to please others perceived to be in power, which is reflected in acquiescence toward the interviewer; (c) accepting the fact that people with ID-DD may require additional time to process the question and formulate a response; and (d) being sensitive to the fact that people with ID-DD may not recall long questions or comprehend complex instructions. Based on these issues, the following interviewing guidelines are critical to the information collection process (Tassé et al., 2005):

- Allow extra time for interviewing the person.

- Introduce yourself and others who are present and indicate the purpose for the interview.

- Encourage the person to invite trusted friends and/or family members to participate in the interview.

- Follow up on responses that suggest the person did not understand the question or the purpose of the interview. This can be done through repeating the request or providing additional examples of personal outcomes or indicators.

- Ask the person to repeat information that the interviewer has not understood.

- If necessary, consult additional resources such as proxies.

Use of Proxies

Personal outcomes can be measured by proxies if the person is unable to respond individually. Before presenting important guidelines regarding the use of proxies, it is important to point out that three procedures used in measuring personal outcomes significantly reduce the need for using proxy respondents: (a) observing and assessing participant behavior using clearly defined behavioral observation measures, (b) simplifying the instructions and response formats, and (c) using self-advocates as trained surveyors (Bonham et al., 2004; Schalock & Bonham, 2003).

We recommend the following five guidelines for use by proxy respondents.

- Proxies should be people who know the individual well.

- Have two people who know the individual well *respond as if they were the person* and then use the *average score* for all subsequent purposes.

- Assessment involving proxies should be clearly identified as another person's perspective.

- As discussed by Stancliffe (2000), the validity of the proxy data must be analyzed in light of the measurement approach used, distinguishing between subjective data obtained from an attitude scale from more objective data. The more objective the indicator, the less discrepancy between the individual's and the proxy's ratings (Verdugo, Schalock, Keith, & Stancliffe, 2005).

- One needs to build the effect of proxy responses into the data analysis. In that regard, Schalock, Bonham, and Marchand (2000) and Bonham et al. (2004) found that proxies: (a) reported higher levels of dignity afforded to the person with disabilities than those who responded for themselves; (b) are more likely than people with disabilities to report greater availability of transportation; and (c) are more likely to underreport QOL scores in the domains of personal development, interpersonal relations, social inclusion, self-determination, and rights; and overreport the quality in physical well-being, emotional well-being, and material well-being.

Figure 3.1 shows the effectiveness of proxies. Our collective experience is that proxies are least effective in assessing subjective QOL indicators (e.g., satisfaction) and defining personal outcomes. Thus in using proxies to measure personal outcomes, all of the above guidelines need to be followed, with additional attention paid to those procedures related to using more objectively based indicators, simplifying the instruction and response formats, and using self-advocates as trained interviewers. Our experience indicates that proxies are most effective in accessing objective indicators (i.e., objective circumstances and experiences), determining what supports are necessary for personal outcomes to occur, determining whether the necessary supports are present, and evaluating whether the supports are effective.

Meeting Psychometric Standards

Historically, quantitative methods have been the principal measurement strategies. But measuring personal outcomes within the QOL context requires the methodological pluralism approach (i.e., quantitative and qualitative) discussed in chapter 1. Meeting psychometric standards is required in both approaches, although the terminology and concepts vary depending on the approach used. This section discusses reliability, validity, and standardization procedures from a more traditional quantitative approach. We then give an overview of four key psychometric standards related to the qualitative approach: credibility, transferability, dependability, and confirmability. Because measuring personal outcomes involves both quantitative and qualitative procedures, personal outcome surveyors should meet both sets of standards. These standards are listed in Table 3.3 and discussed further in chapter 7 within the context of developing indicators at the systems level.

Quantitative Methods

Reliability. Reliability is the extent to which a scale or measure yields a consistent, reproducible measure of performance. There are different types of reliability, and their relevance to the measurement of quality outcomes depends on their use. In reference to individual assessment, *internal consistency reliability* (expressed as Cronbach's alpha; Cronbach, 1951) is frequently used. This type of reliability demonstrates the homogeneity of items or the extent to which the items correlate with one another. For longitudinal (e.g., Time 1 vs. Time 2) comparison, *test-retest reliability* is an essential psychometric property. If proxies are used in the assessment

---

TABLE 3.3

Psychometric Standards Governing the Measurement of Personal Outcomes

---

Quantitative Methods
  Reliability
      Internal consistency (Cronbach's alpha)
      Test-retest
      Interrater
  Validity
      Content
      Construct
      Concurrent
  Standardized procedures
      Survey administration
      Interpretive guidelines
      Data credibility

Qualitative Methods
  Credibility
  Transferability
  Dependability
  Confirmability

---

process, establishing *interrater reliability* is essential. In all cases, reliability coefficients should generally be within the .80 to .85 range for the scale or measure to be considered reliable or consistent.

Validity. Validity is the extent to which a scale or measure assesses what it intends to measure. Currently one finds reference to three types of validity in the individual-referenced QOL literature: content, construct, and concurrent.

Content validity refers to the extent to which the instrument measures the sample of behaviors under consideration. Content validity is shown by demonstrating that the attitude or behaviors measured are consistent with current knowledge. Demonstrating content validity also requires that the items (i.e., indicators and their descriptions) hold up statistically. The two techniques most commonly used for this are Q-sort methodology involving experts in the field (McKeown & Thomas, 1988) and item discrimination, which is the degree to which an item differentiates correctly among respondents in the attitudes and behaviors that the test is designed to measure (Anastasi & Urbina, 1997). The QOL domains and indicators summarized in Tables 2.4–2.7 can be used as a basis for demonstrating content validity.

Construct validity refers to the extent an instrument measures a particular theoretical concept. The construct validity of an instrument is typically demonstrated through

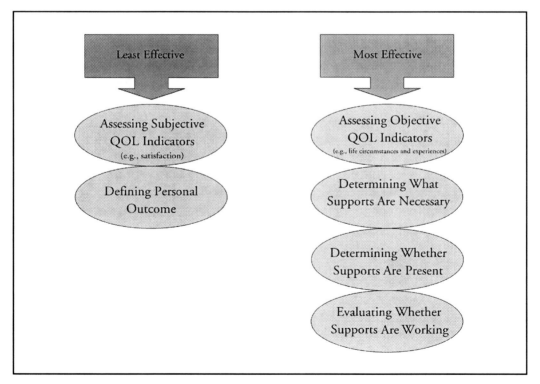

Figure 3.1. Effectiveness of proxies to measure personal outcomes and support needs.

(a) evidence indicating that individuals logically differ on the construct's indicators (e.g., people who are employed should score higher on an employment-related indicator than someone who is unemployed), and (b) factor analysis indicating that the quality domains or their respective indicators represent empirically derived factors. When measuring personal outcomes, an essential element in establishing construct validity is to confirm the factor structure of the QOL model and domains, and demonstrate factor stability across respondent and geographical or cultural groupings (Schalock et al., 2005; Verdugo et al., 2005).

Concurrent validity refers to whether the current scores are consistent with a second, independent measure of the attitude or behavior. This is done typically by correlating scores on two different QOL-related instruments. But due to the current lack of comparable instruments, little research has been done to date on the concurrent validity of quality outcome measures. (The interested reader can find instruments that have been developed to evaluate one's quality of life with varying degrees of demonstrated psychometric properties in Cummins [2004a, 2004b] and Schalock and Verdugo [2002].)

Standardized procedures. Standardized procedures relate to more than simply administering the survey. These important procedures relate to survey administration, interpretive guidelines, and data credibility.

Survey administration is synonymous with interview procedures. An instrument's reliability and validity are enhanced through the use of *standardized procedures*. Such procedures, which are typically included in a standardization manual or set of instructions, include (a) clearly and easily understood definitions of the indicators being measured, (b) clear and easily understood administration directions, (c) clearly defined data collection requirements, (d) procedures for calculating values (i.e., scores), and (e) the intended or appropriate use(s) of the data.

Interpretive guidelines include (a) how to interpret the data, (b) decision-rules regarding their use, (c) clear and easily understood descriptions of data collection strategies, and (d) a discussion of the limitations of the resulting information.

In terms of data credibility, information needs to be available regarding the source of the information, its accuracy, and confirmation that the information corresponds to the respective observation or data-gathering and -reporting period.

Qualitative Standards
Those using qualitative methods to measure personal outcomes also have the responsibility to meet psychometric standards. Although discussed in more detail elsewhere (cf. Schalock, 2001; Schalock & Verdugo, 2002), four relevant standards are (a) *credibility*, which refers to the manner in which the surveyor represents the realities of the participants, and includes techniques such as triangulation, peer debriefing, and member checking; (b) *transferability*, which refers to the extent to which particular findings can be applied to other contexts and other participants,

and includes techniques such as purposeful sampling and describing the methodology and results in considerable detail; (c) *dependability*, which involves an external audit documenting the process by which the survey was conducted; and (d) *confirmability*, which is concerned with objectivity or neutrality and whether someone else looking at the information could trace the conclusions back to the data, understand the logic used to assemble the interpretations into structured coherency, and corroborate the results.

Summary

In summary, it is essential that the instruments or procedure(s) used to measure personal outcomes are reliable and valid, and that standardized procedures are employed. In addition, if individual data are aggregated and used at the organizational or systems level, significant comparison and reporting issues arise. These issues are discussed next.

Methodological Issues in Aggregating Individual Data

Although the primary focus of this chapter is on individual-referenced personal outcomes, one needs to think about their potential use at the organizational or systems level. In this section we discuss methodological issues related to reporting and making judgments based on aggregate data. Related issues will be discussed in chapters 5 and 7.

Reporting Issues

What does one report and use as the basis of aggregation?

In this regard, one issue is whether to use raw scores or standard scores (which are based on a relative position within a distribution of score). Currently raw scores are typically used, due to the lack of quality outcome assessment instruments that provide sufficient data to transform raw scores to standard scores and thus provide an empirically derived distribution of scores. Beyond this lack of data, however, is the more fundamental question and principle regarding the use of comparison in QOL assessments: Should the focus be primarily on the individual or on the person's relative position in a group? Current best practices argue against using personal outcomes for comparative purposes.

A second issue is whether one uses (a) the mean score on the respective indicator or domain, or (b) the proportion of individuals within the respective group expressing the assessed attitude or demonstrating the observed behavior. Currently one finds both being used (see parts 2 & 3). Both raise complex issues regarding comparisons.

Comparison Issues

There are two sensitive and complex issues regarding the use of aggregate data for comparison purposes. The first relates to the unit of comparison—whether it is the person or the group. Conceptually the four measurement principles summarized in Table 3.1 argue strongly for using quality outcomes for individual and program- or performance-enhancement purposes, and not for comparing one person with another.

However, if necessary, our guideline is to use raw score means or proportion of individuals relative to the indicator to make justified comparisons among programs, agencies, or regions. This guideline reflects a number of cautions regarding the use of aggregate data, including (a) by definition, the assessment of quality is subjective, and one cannot define quality for someone else; (b) the principal use of personal outcomes is to enhance personal well-being; (c) one needs to appreciate the complexity of cause-effect relationships between program and individual inputs, processes, and outcomes; and (d) personal outcomes fluctuate greatly over time and situations. Thus the absence of "normative group comparisons" in the field of QOL assessment is no accident.

What comprises the denominator is also a complex comparison issue. Questions arise: For what group of people is this indicator relevant? Are there groups of people who may reasonably experience higher or lower rates of the indicator event? (Karon, Stegemann, & Barnard, 2003). Ideally one wants to use quality indicators that are applicable across all people and that are sensitive to differences in personal attitudes, experiences, and circumstances so that one does not have to change the denominator (referred to frequently as a "risk adjustment"; see chap. 7).

Wrap-Up and Summary

Despite their attractiveness and popularity, the measuring of personal outcomes presents challenges and potential resistance. Most stakeholders have had experiences with and have expectations as to what measurement and "scores" mean. Individuals with disabilities, for example, have typically had a long history of tests and scores that frequently have relegated them to marginal positions in society and reinforced negative stereotypes and stigma. Thus personal outcome measures, which they might equate with IQ tests and mental status evaluations, may be questioned: What is their purpose, intended use, and relevance to enhanced personal well-being? Similarly program staff and administrators frequently question any type of "evaluation" that might be used for funding, certification, monitoring, or enforced change. Thus the emerging emphasis on personal outcomes may be viewed with skepticism and even paranoia. For policy makers and regulators, the issue is similar. Various approaches to enhancing the effectiveness and efficiency of systems-level programs have been attempted in the past and the skeptical people will ask, "What's so different and promising about personal outcomes?"

Thus far in the chapter we have addressed ways to overcome many of those challenges, by having and communicating a clear understanding of the value of measuring outcomes; by understanding and implementing the characteristics of, guidelines for, and principles involved in collecting information; and by successfully mastering four procedural issues, related to interviewing techniques, the use of proxies, meeting psychometric standards, and addressing methodological issues regarding aggregating individual-level data.

In addition, there is considerable published literature on overcoming measurement challenges and potential resistance. Key suggestions, listed in Table 3.4, are based on both our experiences and suggestions found in the published literature (e.g., Dewa, Horgan, Russell, & Keates, 2001; Fox, Kim, & Ehrenkrantz, 2002; Friedman, 2001; Hakes, 2001; Krogh, 1995).

Putting It All Together

The following example demonstrates how one progresses from measuring personal outcomes to using that information to effect quality improvement. It also shows how one service delivery system has met and overcome many of the challenges and potential resistance by using suggestions summarized in Table 3.4. The example is based on the published data associated with the Ask Me! Project in Maryland (Bonham, 2003; Bonham et al., 2004; Schalock & Bonham, 2003).

Overview of Project

The Ask Me! Project, sponsored by the Maryland Developmental Disabilities Administration (DDA) has over the past 6 years developed and standardized an assessment tool to measure quality of life that is based on the eight QOL domains and indicators listed in Table 2.4. The survey uses both subjective and objective quality

---

TABLE 3.4

Suggestions for Overcoming Measurement Challenges and Potential Resistance

---

1. Coordinate well with all stakeholders.

2. Develop successful implementation strategies.

3. Base outcome measuring systems on a broad commitment to customer services and civic mission and instill a commitment to achieve improved performance rather than just a new set of rules.

4. Establish—in consultation with outside overseers—reasonable expectations about what results should and can be measured.

5. Simplify differing existing data collection systems and data collection forms and processes.

6. Use clear definitions and terms.

7. Reduce the burden of data collection through electronic data collection strategies.

8. Explain clearly the purpose of the evaluation and reduce suspicions and mistrust about how the data will be used. Be transparent.

---

indicators. People with developmental disabilities participate in all aspects of the project, including being the primary interviewers during the data collection phase. People with disabilities are also key panelists when the project is presented and results discussed, including discussions as to how the results can be used for programmatic change and improvement.

Primary Focus

Although the primary focus is the individual with developmental disabilities (as reflected in his or her active involvement in the development and selection of quality indicators, role as interviewer, and provider of suggestions regarding how the data can be used to enhance personal well-being), the focus for the personal outcome data is also the organization and the state system. At the organizational level, its primary foci and use are to (a) summarize the assessed QOL scores for program recipients, (b) determine the significant predictors of each of the eight QOL domains, and (c) use this information for staff training and program enhancement. At the systems level, its primary focus and use is on evaluation and systems change based on performance standards.

Principal Data Uses

The 2,200 people interviewed to date in the Ask Me! Project are clustered within 35 providers with about 30 people served by each of the agencies included in the survey to date. The people randomly selected from provider agencies provide estimates of the quality of life of people served by the agencies. The project provides each participating provider with a chart showing how the average quality of life of the people it serves compares to all people supported by DDA, a printout of responses to the individual question by both the people they serve and all those in Maryland, and an electronic spreadsheet with survey responses for each person, unidentified to protect confidentiality. The workshops (which are the first step in the quality improvement process; see below) show providers how to read the data they receive and how other providers have used their information.

The project includes a central quality assurance training session at the beginning of each fall for all participating providers and regional workshops during the year. The training and workshops communicate five topics: (a) the importance that the state places on the quality of life of people it supports, (b) background on QOL concepts and measurement, (c) findings on the quality of life of Marylanders with developmental disabilities, (d) how to read and understand the data agencies receive, and (e) strategies to use the information in program planning and service enhancement. In addition, workshops suggest that providers first compare the average quality of life reported by their clientele to that of all individuals with disabilities in the state and hypothesize reasons why the people they support have higher, lower, or the same scores as the state. If the QOL data do not reflect the goals of the provider, the provider should then ask how it might change its services to best enhance the consumer's quality of life.

A key data set used in program planning and service enhancement is a summary of the factors that statistically relate to (i.e., statistically predict) each of the eight core QOL domains as assessed on the respective core indicators (e.g., the significant predictors of the personal development domain are interpersonal relationships, physical well-being, rights, transportation, and level of cognitive functioning). During the organization-referenced training sessions, administrators and staff are encouraged to think about how programs and services can be developed or changed to enhance these significant predictors and thereby improve the individual's level of personal development and, by inference, personal well-being.

The Maryland DDA uses the data to develop its goals and monitor their achievements as it manages for results—a budget-management requirement of the governor and legislature for all state agencies. The Ask Me! results allow DDA to move beyond the traditional licensing approach to an approach of enhancing quality for all people while maintaining a minimum threshold. Basic to this approach is providing feedback to managers on (a) the predictors of personal development (the initial QOL domain that DDA is focusing on, given the domain's significant relationship to other domains and its consistency with DDA's mission statement); (b) individual-assessed QOL scores; and (c) organizational efforts to meet performance standards. The threshold standard is a positive QOL score (more positive than negative responses to the component questions), and the targets to be maintained or exceeded are the percentage of people with positive scores for each domain at the baseline survey. This threshold ensures that the people whose quality of life is most problematic are not forgotten in the pursuit of enhancing quality of life for all people served. For the first year, DDA set its goal as increasing the average score in the personal development domain by 4%. The goal for the other seven domains is to maintain or increase the average score. DDA does not require individual service providers to use Ask Me! data as they develop quality assurance plans, but encourages its use to measure quality outcomes for all service recipients (Keith & Bonham, 2005).

Summary

The intent of this chapter has not only been to suggest a different way of thinking about measurement and psychometrics, but more specifically to propose a two-component information collection process for measuring personal outcomes. This process involves (a) determining what individuals value based on QOL domains and indicators, and (b) linking that information to the quality improvement process. (In part 3 we discuss how this information can also be linked to other indicators, such as health, welfare, safety, and rights.) To do so, however, requires both an in-person interview and a subsequent placing of the person within the context of community indicators. As we discuss later in chapters 9 and 10, the "quality improvement imperative" is to reduce the discrepancy between personal outcomes and community QOL indicators. Thus, although we cannot have norms on how people define outcomes, we can measure whether people achieve their personal outcomes and thus move toward the community.

Measuring personal outcomes requires a different approach to measurement (as just discussed) and also a number of challenges to organizations and systems. These relate to the four key procedural issues discussed: interviewing techniques, the use of proxies, meeting psychometric standards, and overcoming complex issues regarding the aggregation of individual data for use at the organizational and systems level. In addition to these challenges, readers should be aware that measured personal outcomes are only one's best approximation to the reality and complexity of the person's life. Thus one needs to remember that (a) personal outcome scores should be considered as relative and not absolute; (b) gain scores are potentially problematic, because one's subjective evaluation of life conditions may reflect a trait more than a changing external condition; (c) the potential ceiling effect may preclude longitudinal comparisons; (d) one's perception of quality changes over time, therefore one should expect only incremental changes; (e) the relative importance of quality indicators (and thus personal outcomes) will vary across the life span of the person and among cultures; and (f) the assessment of quality outcomes requires a commitment to longitudinal measurement and evaluation.

As stressed throughout the chapter, quality indicators and personal outcomes extend beyond the person to the organization, the system, and the community. It is to the organizational level that we now turn, as we discuss in part 2 the organizational perspective, focusing on management strategies, examples of the integration and synthesis of different valued outcomes by the service or support providers, and the evolving role of service and provider organizations to connect people with their communities.

PART 2

The Organizational Perspective

Because they affect both the lives of consumers and the anticipated activities of organizations, personal outcomes cannot be viewed in isolation. How organizations approach and use personal outcomes is the focus of this part of the text.

In chapter 4 we discuss the challenges involved in organizations transitioning to more individualized, dispersed support systems and the practices that contribute to the successful management of the organization from a personal outcomes, quality of life (QOL) perspective. We describe a management and leadership strategy that opens the organizational doors inward to enable people, including those receiving supports, staff, and volunteers, and families and the community, to understand their own strengths, resources, and unique capabilities. The chapter builds on what we know about social capital, organizational processes that facilitate personal outcomes, leadership models and organizational culture, human resource development strategies, the community as a resource, and how to nurture and sustain healthy organizations. The chapter also discusses the requirements for managing for outcomes: self-advocate leadership and decision making; competent leadership style; and constant measurement, communication, and reinforcement for organizational processes that facilitate personal outcomes.

Chapter 5 summarizes the Council on Quality and Leadership's (1997, 2000d, 2005b) *Personal Outcome Measures,* including their development, validation, and use for quality improvement. The chapter also explores emerging trends in the definition, measurement, and use of personal outcome measures. Although person-centered planning and the metrics of person-centered outcomes have focused attention on the individual, there is growing evidence to suggest that we need to shift attention to individuals and their supports in the context of community-oriented definitions, measurement, and applications of personal quality of life. The research and practices related to social capital, community QOL indicators, and social change suggest a shift in focus from organizational quality improvement to community quality of life for all citizens.

If such a shift is to occur, a number of current concepts need to be reexamined. Chief among these are the concept of disability, quality of life as a community variable, the definition and major components of social capital as applied to individuals with disabilities, the role of organizations, and the relationships among individuals, organizations, and communities.

Throughout these two chapters, the reader is encouraged to think seriously about three things. First, we ask that you think about your own quality of life and how you define and measure personal outcomes, and how your organization's services and support activities influence the personal outcomes of your service recipients. Second, consider the importance to individuals with intellectual and developmental disabilities of the concepts discussed in these two chapters, including values, person-centered planning, personal outcome measurement, basic health and welfare assurances, and organizational performance. Third, think also about the role that one's community can play in enhancing both the quality of services provided to people with intellectual and developmental disabilities and the enhanced personal outcomes resulting from those services.

CHAPTER 4

Managerial Strategies: Opening the Doors Inward

Introduction and Overview

The quality of life (QOL) construct and its measurement through personal outcomes has challenged traditional forms of management in disability organizations. Organizations are changing program and service models that were based on standardization, uniformity, and predictability into systems of supports and opportunities based on individualization, differences, and uniqueness. Static programs, such as the group home, sheltered workshop, employment training, or transitional living, are evolving into integrated community supports. In addition, integrated disability services are being incorporated into community life supports for all citizens, merging with the developing social dynamic of inclusive communities. The discussion of quality and quality of life is moving beyond the boundaries of individual service and support organizations.

This link between inclusive communities and QOL definition and measurement is reshaping our thinking about supports to people with intellectual and developmental disabilities (ID-DD). Individuality and self-directedness are increasing as the prevalence of centrally directed, uniform, and consistent programs decrease. Managing this emerging community support system requires very different skills.

Large formal systems of service are managed from a mechanistic frame; they are designed for repetition and productivity and to support a limited range of choice and options within an identified program or set of services. These mechanistic systems are not designed for problem solving, innovation, and adaptation within inclusive communities; nor are they designed for people (rather than programs) to make choices. In contrast, small, less formal organizations are based on an organic model that emphasizes adaptation, innovation, individual responsiveness, and less repetition of uniform processes (Gardner, 1995, 2002).

This transition from the formal, centralized service system to a more individualized and dispersed support system presents seeming contradictions. Successful management of the process requires constant attention to, and balancing of, opposing pressures. Delegation of authority requires feedback. Decentralization of authority requires local autonomy, authority, and capability. Offering people choices and opportunities increases the possibility of financial inefficiency, less adherence to defined procedures, and greater variability of employee performance. Peters and Waterman (1982) referred to this dynamic as "simultaneous loose-tight properties." Capra (1991) described this as the "interplay of ying and yang," the constant interplay of polar opposites that govern the change process.

Nonprofit leaders cannot escape or avoid these apparent contradictions. Rather, they learn to cope, live with, and manage the pressure. In addition, they teach and model the management of this dynamic interaction for organizational employees. Vail (1993) used the metaphor of a still, tranquil pond at the bottom of a dangerous series of rapids as the hoped-for place of rest, solace, and reflection for those leaders who withstood the journey down the stream. But, Vail concludes, there is no tranquil pond; for the effective manager, there is only an ongoing passage through the white water of change and contradiction.

The purpose of this chapter is to discuss the challenges of organizations transitioning to more individualized, dispersed support systems. The chapter also presents managerial practices that open the organizational doors inward to enable all stakeholders to understand their own strengths, resources, and capabilities. The chapter begins by asking, What characterizes organizations managing for change? It progresses to a discussion of suggested practices that make personal outcome systems work. These practices are categorized in terms of strategy, execution, culture, structure, and leadership.

What Characterizes Organizations Managing for Change?

Organizations have developed many different strategies for addressing challenges related to decentralization, self-directed supports inclusion, and managing change. Some organizations demonstrate creativity and resolve; others reject the challenge and the need for change. Reger, Gustafson, DeMarie, and Mullane (1994) suggest that employees may reject the need for change because their beliefs about the organization's identity create cognitive opposition to fundamental change. The authors identify three alternative probabilities for change acceptance.

First, the change is perceived as *unnecessary:* "We're already doing that. Our mission and values include personal outcomes, self-determination, and community inclusion." Employees perceive no gap between values and vision and current organizational performance.

Second, the change is perceived as *unobtainable:* "Those values and visions are fine, but too unrealistic for us. We're not funded to do that; the regulations won't allow us to do that; our workforce can't implement that; the people we support are really unique and those ideas won't work here." The gap between current performance and the vision and values is perceived as too great. There are two variations of unobtainable. The first is "not now" or "we're preparing" or "we need to fix a problem before we worry about quality." Thus organization waits until the new board members are elected, until after the legislature adjourns, or until some defined event takes place. In some cases organizations hide out and escape from action in planning exercises. The second variation of "unobtainable" is financial inability to make organizations work. As the federal and state governments alter funding mechanisms and payment rates, more and more nonprofits are experiencing financial distress.

Third, the change is perceived as a *worthy and legitimate challenge:* "We recognize the challenge, and believe we have the leadership. We believe that all people can succeed with the right supports. The employees can meet the challenge." The organization believes it can bridge the gap between current and future performance. It recognizes the gap between vision and values and current practice, but it is challenged to narrow the gap.

The successful organization defines and frames the change process within a range of perceived do-ability. The change is not seen as so slight that employees fail to grasp its significance; nor is the change seen as so radical as to be unacceptable.

Management theory and practice offers organizations alternatives in reframing cognitive impediments to change and altering organizational leadership, culture, and performance to promote change. However, the purpose of this chapter is to explore the practices that contribute to the successful management of the organization from a personal outcome, QOL perspective. This, then, leads to a second question: What are the critical success factors in making a personal outcome system work?

What Really Works?

Personal outcome systems work when leaders integrate the values and content of personal outcomes with or within key managerial processes. The two parts of a successful QOL personal outcome system are organizational values and competence. In that regard, like the models for person-directed planning (Newton & Horner, 2004) and appreciative inquiry (Busche, 1998; Cooperrider & Srivastva, 1987), organizations need to build change around their own strengths. This internal analysis is as important as the knowledge of other models, programs, experiences, tools, techniques, and successful approaches in other organizations, communities, or states.

Joyce, Nohira, and Roberson (2003) have recently addressed the question of *What Really Works* in regard to the managerial practices that produce superior results for American business organizations. They write:

For years we have watched new management ideas come and go, passionately embraced one year, abruptly abandoned the next. "What really works?" we wondered. . . . Our finding took us quite by surprise. Most of the management tools and techniques we studied had no direct causal relationship to superior business performance. What does matter, it turns out, is having a strong grasp of the business basics. (p. 43)

Thus the critical success factor in making a personal outcome system work is a strong grasp of the business basics—in our world, of the value-based, not-for-profit, community-based support system. These nonprofit business basics are located, examined, and improved by opening the door inward and exploring organizational management for outcomes. As in the world of business and commerce, the basic managerial practices of strategy, execution, culture, and structure will determine the success of our personal outcome, QOL initiatives for people with ID-DD.

Values, beliefs, and principles are prerequisites to the successful facilitation of personal outcomes for people, but by themselves they are insufficient. Organizations won't succeed in facilitating personal outcomes without management and leadership capability.

The remaining sections of this chapter approach the management of personal outcomes from the framework suggested by Joyce and colleagues—that there are a core set of managerial factors that account for organizational success. We will focus on the following five factors, as shown in Figure 4.1: (a) strategy—a plan or method based on values and vision; (b) execution—the performance of the plan or method; (c) culture—the bond that unites and energizes people in execution; (d) structure—

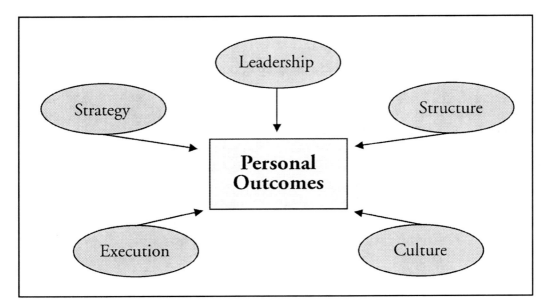

Figure 4.1. Organizational factors that enhance personal outcomes.

roles, relationships, reporting, and feedback mechanisms that support culture; and (e) leadership—initiative and energy exercised by people, individually and collectively, throughout the structure. In subsequent sections we will discuss how each of these factors can promote improved-quality personal outcomes for people with ID-DD in a wide range of formal and informal organizations.

Strategy

In this context, strategy is defined as the integration of vision, mission, and values within an action plan designed to produce identified outcomes. One's organizational strategy must be built around a clear value proposition for the primary customer. This requires a clear understanding of, and commitment to, the people with ID-DD receiving services and supports. Organizations, formal or informal, public or private, large or small, often involve multiple stakeholders. For small, self-help support organizations, these stakeholders can include friends, volunteers, family members, and people with disabilities. More formal organizations may involve additional stakeholders, such as funders, regulators, boards of directors.

Successful strategy begins with the clear definition of the person with the disability as the primary customer. Organizations need to carefully identify both the assumptions and implications of this position. Defining the value proposition for the primary customer within the context of organization (either formal or informal) requires time, patience, and clarity of purpose. Organizations need to reach consensus on the values and assumptions that both support individuals and guide organizations. Organizations need to balance their "loose-tight properties" at both the individual and organizational levels. This balance determines financial, emotional, and social complexity of the organization and raises two questions: (a) What role will people with disabilities play in the leadership and governance of the organization? (b) How will we prepare all stakeholders for this role?

Strategy Initiatives
Successful strategy for increasing quality of life for people with disabilities is based on three focused initiatives: social capital, bridging organizations, and personal outcomes. These three initiatives, shown in Figure 4.2, singularly and collectively define and then translate vision, mission, and values into action plans.

Social Capital
Social capital refers to the bonds of trust and reciprocity that develop between individuals (Coleman, 1994; Putnam, 2000). Social capital is an asset. Consider that both financial capital (money in the bank) and human resource capital (education, skills, and experiences) can be used to secure goods, services, and a quality of life as we might each define it. The same is true for social capital.

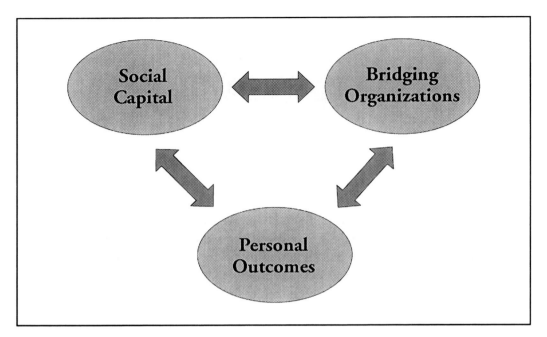

Figure 4.2. Quality of life strategy initiatives.

Relationships of trust and reciprocity enable us to use our social capital for supports, favors, access to other social networks; to find jobs, locate new friends, and find allies and advocates to stand up for us when our interests are threatened. The research on the impact of social capital on individual welfare is worldwide and consistent. Social capital increases positive outcomes in our psychological, physical, social, and financial well-being. This wide-ranging impact of social capital is particularly important for people with disabilities, because they often lack financial capital and human resource capital.

Social capital is a common bond for networks that connect all people within a community. Social capital is both a perquisite for inclusive communities and a major determinant of quality of life. More important, however, social capital applies to all stakeholders involved in the provision of supports and services. One's organizational strategy of building social capital applies to organizational staff and volunteers, families, and neighborhood and community representatives. Successful organizations link the networks of people with disabilities and their families with the networks of employees, volunteers, their families, friends, neighbors, and community members. The interlocking web of social capital networks results in inclusive communities.

Bridging Organizations
The phrase *bridging organizations* refers to the primary function of service and support organizations. The role of organizations is not simply to provide services and supports.

Rather, the mission of the organization is to use service and support resources to connect people with and within their own communities.

This definition of the organization *as a bridge to the community* for people with ID-DD is a departure from the traditional function of the disability organization. As a bridge, an organization represents a means to the end of community inclusion, rather than as an end in itself as a continuing provider of services and supports. Organizations as bridges:

- Define transitional and changing roles for themselves. Their roles and responsibilities become as varied as the people and the communities they try to link. Some traditional providers may no longer be operating workshops, group homes, or developmental training programs, but many people with intellectual disabilities will need ongoing assistance with financial management, health care, individual therapy, and basic self-help skills.

- Play a continuous bridging role in connecting people to the community.

- Display organic characteristics as they balance the dynamics of self-directed services with the evolving quality of community life. The responsive organization adapts its bridging structures and process to optimize the fit between community life and people with ID-DD.

The strategy that incorporates the initiatives of social capital and bridging must clearly articulate the voice and message of the organization's primary customer, as the message relates to the individual meaning that each person gives to his or her priority outcome. This person-centered strategy will be found in the individual meaning that each person gives to his or her priority outcomes. Thus each person's definition of the personal outcomes (e.g., choosing work, having friends, being safe) drives organizational strategy.

Personal Outcomes

Personal outcomes provide the values, organizational methodology, and metrics for implementing and evaluating the successes of our social capital and organizational bridging initiatives. As discussed more fully in chapter 5, the application of the personal outcomes results in (a) the development of a person-directed plan of individually defined priorities that identifies one's valued outcomes; (b) the development of an organizational strategy and the supports to facilitate the valued outcomes—a clear challenge to the organization to facilitate those outcomes by creatively formulating needed supports; and (c) a measurement methodology to determine the success of facilitating those priority outcomes while simultaneously enhancing basic assurances in the area of health, safety, and human security.

Strategy Implementation

Strategy includes communication within the organization and to external stakeholders.

In effect, the ongoing communication of the mission, vision, and values is the strategy. Effective strategy requires ongoing, consistent, and pervasive communication along four different channels within the organization and outward to the community: stories, positions and tasks, employee development, and the planning process.

Stories

The stories that people tell in organizations convey meaning about values, heroes, and expectations. Successful strategy uses stories to convey meaning, about people achieving outcomes, staff and volunteers supporting people in achieving outcomes, and families and communities affirming the importance of outcomes. Organizational heroes, the protagonists in the stories, are those people who enable others to accumulate social capital, cross bridges into the community, and facilitate personal outcomes for others.

Stories are conveyed in multiple forms. People with disabilities use stories to describe their past. They can also use stories to convey their dreams and hopes for the future. Organizations use stories to describe learning about and facilitating outcomes for people. As such, they become part of the planning process. Stories also support formal and informal celebrations. People rejoice, relive, and enjoy the stories about personal outcome attainment.

Sometimes stories stretch the truth, and people are transformed into heroes. This exaggeration indicates the importance of the attributes attached to the hero. Successful strategy often creates heroes to highlight the values and actions attributed to the hero. Bridges and bridge builders have often served as cultural icons in United States history (Tractenberg, 1965). Our human service organizations should do no less in assigning a hero's status to the very best bridge builders.

Stories can also be expressed in writing and in video to convey the meaning of personal outcomes to other stakeholders. The combination of personal outcome data, art or photography, and individual stories is a particularly powerful combination in conveying meaning to community representatives, funders, and legislators.

Position Descriptions and Task Assignments

Employees and volunteers generally demonstrate performance that follows expectations established by the organization. Strategy requires that organizations link position descriptions, employee or volunteer performance evaluations, and task assignments with personal outcome attainment. The position description and task assignments become a bridge that carries the action strategy of personal outcome attainment throughout the organization.

Position descriptions and evaluation clearly indicate that the organization and its employees and volunteers are focused on building social capital for all organizational members and connecting its organizational members to their communities. Success in these two initiatives will be reflected in personal outcomes attainment.

Orientation and Employee or Volunteer Development

Effective strategy includes initial orientation and subsequent employee and volunteer training and development that is linked to person-centered outcomes. Organizational rules, informal practices, policy, procedure, and protocol are explained within the context of facilitating personal outcomes for people with ID-DD. Organizational training, personal and career development initiatives, and ongoing in-service educational offerings are clearly connected and defined in terms of promoting personal outcomes.

The Planning Process

Most funding and regulatory authorities require some form of plan that includes resource allocation information. The form and requirement of this document (e.g., individual education plan, individual habilitation plan, individual written rehabilitation plan, individual program plan, individual service plan) clearly connect goals, objectives, and methods to individually identified personal outcome measures.

This planning process requires a defined sequence in supporting people to achieve their personal outcomes. The first step in the planning process is to identify and define the individual's priority personal outcomes. This provides a context or rationale for targeting those functional or clinical outcomes that will facilitate personal outcomes. The relationship among the personal, functional, and clinical outcomes is presented in Table 4.1.

This strategic sequencing of outcomes does not mean that functional and/or clinical outcomes are not important; rather, functional and clinical outcomes greatly increase in importance when we realize that those outcomes facilitate the individually defined personal outcomes. This identification and prioritization of personal outcomes defines

TABLE 4.1 Outcome Design Index™				
Outcome	Definition Focus	Result	Measure	Measurement
Personal	Dreams and priorities	Life fulfillment	Personal outcomes	Multiple samples of one
Functional	Life functions	Increased capacity	Functional scales	Norms and median scores
Clinical	Symptoms	Symptom reduction	Cure, remission	Charts, records, utilization review

Note. From *Challenging Tradition: Measuring Quality Through Personal Outcomes* (p. 10), by J. F. Gardner, 2003, Towson, MD: Council on Quality in Leadership. Copyright 2003 by Council on Quality and Leadership. Reprinted with permission.

personal quality of life, guides organizational goal setting and resource allocation, and ultimately mobilizes families, friends, and communities on behalf of people with ID-DD. Increasing functional capabilities or clinical outcomes as ends in themselves is no longer sufficient. Acquiring skills that cannot be generalized or enhancing health status in segregated settings is insufficient. Quality of life requires that we use medical science, teaching skills, and habilitation and rehabilitation methodology to increase clinical and functional outcomes that facilitate each individual's personal outcomes within the context of inclusive communities.

Execution

For our purposes, execution is defined as disciplined, consistent, and flawless management and enactment of strategy. Execution begins with the person's own definition and meaning of his or her personal outcomes, moves to the organization's design and delivery of the supports to facilitate the personal outcomes, and continues in the ongoing measurement of personal outcome attainment at the individual and aggregate level.

For these three functions to be successful, the organization must deliver on its strategic value proposition for people with ID-DD and keep its word, doing what it says it will do. Self-determination means self-determination. Choosing where to live and work really means choosing a home and job. The organization must also deliver on its promise to other stakeholders, whether they are families, employees, volunteers, or the community. Recognizing that there are often conflicts and trade-offs among stakeholders, organizations must be guarded in the commitments and promises they make to the full range of stakeholders. Optimally organizations make limited, but important, promises to their stakeholders and then deliver on those commitments.

Successful execution involves five key actions: (a) incorporating the best methods and sound science, (b) giving decision-making responsibility to direct-support professionals, (c) avoiding unnecessary routines, (d) making personal outcome measurement constant and pervasive, and (e) communicating values, expectations, and measurement.

Incorporate the Best Methods and Sound Science

The principles of self-directed services and the values found in the personal outcomes are derived from feedback from people with ID-DD. They have their own definitions of quality of life. The pursuit of QOL outcomes requires that we approach each individual as a unique sample of one. Each person has his or her own definition of each of the personal outcomes. This uniqueness means that (a) each person may define outcomes differently, and the priority outcomes will vary over time, and (b) the supports needed for one person naming a particular outcome may be significantly different from supports needed for another person naming the same outcome. Because of differing definitions for an outcome, a variety of methods to facilitate that outcome may be needed within a single organization. The methods that successfully facilitate outcomes for one person may be inappropriate for another.

Good execution requires that we identify transferable methods and sound science from best-practice models, demonstration projects, and other benchmarked methods. Successful models, demonstration projects, and data-based practices offer guidelines on how to construct bridges to the community for people served. However, the bridges must be built on the terrain of the local community and involve individualized supports.

Research from the field of dissemination of innovation (Rogers, 1995) indicates that most organizations reinvent best practice and model demonstrations. Rogers defined reinvention as "the extent to which an innovation is changed or modified by a user in the process of its adoption and implementation" (p. 174). Organizations can identify the generalizable or transferable aspects of best-practice models, and, by opening their own doors inward, decide what can best be applied in their own situations.

Give Decision-Making Responsibility to Direct-Support Professionals

Using person-directed QOL measures to determine, plan, and facilitate personal outcomes requires an ongoing dialogue. This dialogue takes place every day between and among people with disabilities and the staff and volunteers who support them. Experiences, both daily and long term, will alter the meaning of the outcomes and require changes in support strategies.

This ongoing, iterative process is different from the traditional assessment and service planning model that unfolds according to scheduled assessments, reports, reviews, and meetings. What is called "personal outcomes QOL engagement" means that direct-support professionals have the capacity and authority to discover changes in the meanings of personal outcomes and revise daily and interactive supports to facilitate changed outcomes. The discovery and facilitation of personal outcomes is best accomplished in real time by families, friends, staff, and volunteers. The creative use of formal and informal community resources to promote personal outcomes requires people who are connected to their communities. They are able to use organizational resources to connect people to social capital networks and community opportunities.

Avoid Unnecessary Routines

Services and supports organized around program models often generate an overabundance of policies, procedures, and expectations for proscribed behaviors from all stakeholders. Many of these habits and behaviors, however, do not support individually defined QOL outcomes. Organizations can work backward from defined outcomes to identify and then eliminate those organizational practices that no longer facilitate personal outcomes. Key questions for execution: (a) Why are we engaging in this activity? (b) How does this routine, requirement, or activity facilitate people's personal outcomes?

Make Personal Outcome Measurement Constant and Pervasive

Organizations use personal outcome data and analysis to answer the question: How well are we doing? The answer to the question is found in both the data measuring personal outcomes and, more important, the organization's analysis and use of the data. The meaning attached to the personal outcome data informs decision making and increases accountability throughout the organization. Measuring personal outcomes can include the following components:

- Routinely defining and redefining people's definitions of their priority outcomes. This feedback takes place on a day-to-day basis.

- Regularly applying the outcome measurement methodology to determine the status of individual attainment as well as the aggregate analysis of outcomes for specific people and for the whole organization. This is often accomplished on an annual or semiannual basis.

- Validating the ongoing personal outcome measurement by designated staff or volunteers, external interviewers, or other personnel. These validation interviews offer an opportunity to test the regular measurement and interpretation of data analysis. The validation reviews often serve as case studies for organizational improvement.

- Holding open-book meetings (Stack, 1992) on a regular basis that feature the organization's learning and knowledge about personal outcome attainment and the effectiveness of the individualized supports and services provided by the organization. These meetings discuss the organization's measurement and performance analysis. During the meetings employees establish base-line and target outcome levels for the organization. They also report measurement that provides the objective criteria to support story telling and hero development, performance evaluations for staff and volunteers, celebrations, accountability documentation for other stakeholders, and staff training and orientation.

Communicate Values, Expectations, and Measurement

Successful organizations constantly communicate their values and cultural priorities, expectations for staff and volunteers, and organizational results. Successful organizations proceed on the assumption that basic messages must be focused and repeated due to constant turnover, daily turmoil and distractions, and competing messages arising from both formal and informal sources within the organization. The constant communication of the basic values surrounding personal outcome measures, self-directed services, and quality of life for all people must be repeated on a daily basis. The language of personal outcomes is incorporated into all formal and informal communication.

Values are best communicated through a combination of pictures, stories, and data. Each mode of communication reinforces the other. The pictures present a visual image to which the observer responds. The narrative tells the story behind the picture and provides the context and perspective for interpretation. The data on personal outcomes connects the person and his or her story with the organization's success in facilitating outcomes for people.

Culture

In managerial parlance, culture is the bonding and glue that unites and energizes people in the execution of strategy. Deal and Kennedy (1999) suggest that culture is a power lever that guides organizational behavior. More specifically, a strong culture is a system of informal rules that spells out how people are to behave most of the time, and thus enables people to feel better about what they do, so they are more likely to work harder.

Successful organizations develop a culture that stresses the importance of making personal outcomes happen for each person receiving services and supports. This culture of high performance goes beyond a commitment to values and principles. The organization stresses personal outcome attainment. The strong culture results in an acceleration of attainment rather than progress at a consistent velocity.

This culture, grounded in execution and values-based strategy, incorporates the belief that successful personal outcome attainment is the only leadership option for the organization. Once staff and volunteers have identified people's outcomes through ongoing interviews and dialogues, the only barrier to facilitating the outcome is found in people's creativity, imagination, and unexplored community resource networks. The limitation to personal outcome achievement is found not in the individual definition of the outcome, but rather in the organization's inability to creatively search for, and build bridges to, alternative support solutions. In addition, an organizational culture based on the personal outcomes QOL engagement emphasizes: (a) mindful thinking, (b) organizational anchors, (c) linking performance with rewards, and (d) making work personal.

Mindful Thinking

Langer (1997) uses the phrase *creative inability* to mean an inability to respond to new signals. In contrast, she defines a *mindful approach* as the "continuous creation of new categories, openness to new information, and an implicit awareness of more than one perspective" (p. 4). The individual's definition of his or her priority outcome is a "new signal." The needed supports are often found not in the categories of existing programs, but rather in social capital networks, in organizational creativity, and along the bridges of community opportunity.

Organizations expand the range of available supports when they break down personal outcome definitions into interests (i.e., outcomes or ends) and positions (i.e., strategies or means). Fisher and Ury (1988) noted that any successful negotiation begins with identification of an interest rather than a single position that satisfies that interest. Relating this to personal outcomes, practitioners attempt to understand the client's interest in the definition of his or her outcome. This distinction between interests and positions enables support staff to identify the reasons why (i.e., interests) a person might want to live on Brookwood Road or work at Chase Pitken Gardens. Then the support staff can identify a range of residential or employment options that address the person's interests. For example, one might initially choose Brookwood Road because of the type of home; its proximity to transportation, friends, family, or work; or its reputation as a safe neighborhood. Once the interests are identified, there may well be other locations that can accommodate those interests. Rather than get locked into a decision about whether "Brookwood Road is reasonable," the questions shifts to what other locations will satisfy the interests.

Thus mindful thinking is that part of an organization's culture that encourages multiple perspectives and approaches built on the client's expressed interests and personal outcomes. Acting on those interests and desired outcomes requires the collective action of people with the responsibility and authority to act—that is, organizational anchors.

Organizational Anchors

Self-directed services result from the collective action of people with the responsibility and authority to make and carry out decisions. People receiving services and supports need information, opportunities and experience in decision making, and people who will support them in their decision experiences. Staff and volunteers providing individualized supports need the skills, abilities, and the authorization to design and provide supports that facilitate outcomes for people. As much as possible, an organizational culture that promotes self-direction and QOL outcomes places maximum authority and responsibility on direct-support professionals.

With the delegation of authority and responsibility, organizations must also provide direct-support professionals with the following: (a) training in the design and provision of supports; (b) policies, procedures, and guidelines that enable them to make informed decisions consistent with organizational values and polity; (c) technical assistance and consultation from senior staff in analyzing and making decisions that involve dilemmas, ethical considerations, and difficult decisions about competing values; and (d) opportunities and supports to achieve their own personal outcomes.

Collectively, the organizational vision, values, training, policy, and procedures serve as anchors for staff and volunteers. Strong anchors keep organizational practice and individual behaviors within a defined area of individual and collective discretion. Staff and volunteers exercise creativity, managers support innovative alternatives, and families and friends develop confidence in the support options when they recognize that the system is anchored in strong foundations of health, safety, and human security.

The values, vision, policies, and procedures that serve as anchors for staff and volunteer initiatives are designed for clients in the middle of the bell-shaped curve, where behaviors and responses are consistent and predictable. Too often, because of failures to provide basic assurances in the past, organizations design policies and procedures around the "outliers" at the ends of the bell-shaped curve, people whose behaviors, health, and human security needs are unpredictable and often extreme. The effect is to overly restrict staff and volunteer initiative (and often the rights and opportunities of other people) because of the behaviors of the outlier population. Effectively anchored policies and procedures allow staff to identify and support outliers and still use judgment and creativity in facilitating personal outcomes for others (Schalock & Luckasson, 2005).

Link Performance With Rewards

Successful organizations establish and reinforce a culture of person-directed QOL outcomes by rewarding performance linked to those outcomes. We have noted that successful organizations build organizational strategy on a linkage between position descriptions, hiring criteria, performance evaluations, and promotion. Organizations then reward this successful linkage with financial incentives. The financial incentives work at several levels. At the time of distribution, the monetary value of the reward is particularly important. In addition, the accumulated monetary rewards and increase in salary may increase the retention rates of the valued employees. Flannery, Hofrichter, and Platten (1996) note that "compensation must inextricably be tied to people, their performance, and the organization vision and values that their performance supports" (p. 4).

However, most organizations face limits in offering monetary rewards. Alternative forms of recognition, ranging from informal verbal feedback to more involved employee recognition programs, special events, and celebrations, can help to build a culture of self-directed supports and person-centered quality of life. Many organizations have discovered a link between retention of valued employees and a culture that stresses celebration, recognizes employee contributions, provides recognition and reinforcement, and, most important, provides direct supervisory feedback to the direct-support professional.

Make This Work Personal

In an organization where personal outcomes are the central value, employees and volunteers find similarities between the pursuit of their own personal outcomes and their support for other people. They are challenged to facilitate outcomes for others because they understand the importance of their own personal outcomes. Personal outcomes take on a very personal meaning. An organizational culture that defines work in terms of facilitating personal outcomes offers staff far greater challenges than defining work in terms of a tasks, duties, and responsibilities.

Structure

Organizational structure includes the formal roles, relationships, and reporting and feedback mechanisms that enable the culture to execute strategy. Robbins (1990) defines structure as the manner in which tasks are allocated, who reports to whom, and the methods of communication and coordination within the organization. Providing services and supports for people with ID-DD requires a grounding in vision and values as well as organizational policy and procedure. Good organizational anchors translate these into clear definitions of staff and volunteer roles and responsibilities. Policy and procedure should offer guidance for action rather than barriers to initiative. Neither should increase complexity or layers of reporting.

However, most nonprofit and human service organizations are mission driven and not market focused. As such, rules, policies, and procedures accumulate and build up over time. New organizational requirements and processes are often added on top of existing procedures. Similarly public sectors at the federal, state, and local levels pass new legislation, enact new regulations, and implement new requirements but seldom sweep the old and unused requirements off the books. Thus, in thinking about structure as one of the five critical factors for a personal outcome system, the reader is encouraged to consider: (a) designing services with as little management as possible, (b) promoting the exchange of knowledge, (c) connecting thinking and doing, and (d) bridging to the community.

Minimizing Management

Human service and other nonprofit organizations can manage the slow creep of added procedural requirements by stressing simplicity. This is particularly important for organizations (a) that are employee- and volunteer-labor intensive, (b) that serve other people, and (c) in which the needs and interests of the people often require organizational flexibility. Bardach (1977) summarized this challenge with the admonition that organizations design services that require as "little management as possible." He noted that "programs predicated on continuing high levels of competence, on expeditious interorganizational coordination, or sophisticated methods . . . are very vulnerable" (p. 253). More recently Trout and Rivkin (1999) have offered a similar observation using the large symphony orchestra as the metaphor. In the orchestra, he notes, there are no vice conductors or other intermediaries between the conductor and the symphony members. There is only one conductor and one musical score to guide the many different musicians.

Promoting the Exchange of Knowledge and Information

Promoting the exchange of knowledge and information requires a mix of cultural and structural factors. Human service organizations are rich in *tacit knowledge*—knowledge that has been developed and internalized by organizational members over extended periods of time. Direct-support professionals acquire this tacit knowledge from their daily interaction with people they support. They know and understand the people they support, but they often find it difficult to capture this knowledge in reports, narratives, or data summaries. The communication of tacit information requires trust, a common culture, and the use of stories, narrative, and art. Organizational structures must provide the opportunity for the exchange of tacit information.

In contrast, *explicit knowledge* can be more easily captured, summarized, and disseminated. Staff does this through reports, data analysis, assessments, or meeting summaries (Davenport & Prusak, 1998; Nonaka & Takeuchi, 1995). Organizational structures must be consistent with organizational culture and support the communication of explicit information. The cultural values must reinforce the organizational behaviors of collecting, analyzing, sharing, and using new and existing information. This cultural requirement is a necessary foundation for any level of explicit-information exchange within the organization (Zuboff, 1988). Without the organizational culture promoting and encouraging knowledge acquisition and exchange, it makes little difference whether information systems rely on "word of mouth," staff entries in daily logs and records, or automated digital systems. What matters is that knowledge and information exchange be useful, support the attainment of personal outcomes, and contribute to quality enhancement within the organization.

"White-water" or crisis management will succeed only if sufficient methods for information feedback and organizational responsiveness are already in place. Management science has demonstrated that decentralization and delegation require monitoring systems (Robbins, 1990). In community-based support systems, an information-feedback system must be flexible, practical, and meaningful to support the system, direct-services professionals, and volunteers. Information collection and analysis, and action based on that information, should be ongoing and regularly scheduled. Dash board indicators, such as unusual incident reports and priority medical and behavioral monitoring, may take place daily. Other information, such as staff usage patterns, vendor payments, retirement, and health insurance payments, and personal outcome measure information, is collected on a regular basis but generally analyzed on a monthly or quarterly basis by senior managers. Such information feedback will enhance organizational responsiveness.

Connecting Thinking and Doing

Traditional structures identify "thinkers" as senior managers at the top or center of the organizational picture. The "doers," who implement management decisions, are typically located at the bottom or periphery of the organization. In bureaucratic structures the separation of thinkers from doers reinforces a lack of feedback and prevents the transfer of tacit knowledge. Facilitating personal outcomes, in contrast, requires direct-support professionals to take responsibility for simultaneously thinking and doing. Direct-support professionals link the client with the supports that will facilitate an outcome, and they provide feedback to all stakeholders on the attainment of the outcomes and/or the possible redefinition of the outcome.

Progressive organizations encourage direct-support professionals to stay engaged with people receiving services and supports and to link thinking and doing. This expands their authority without necessarily making them managers. Organizations develop structures that facilitate this interaction as they encourage direct-support professionals to develop skills, enhance performance, and yet stay connected to clients. Staff and volunteers have the opportunity to develop new skills and abilities in problem solving, negotiating, and conflict resolution, but they also stay engaged in communicating tacit knowledge, translating it into explicit knowledge, and facilitating personal outcomes.

Bridging to the Community

The structure of a service-oriented organization serves as a bridge between the community and the people served. As such, the quality of community life influences the type and intensity of support available for facilitating the personal outcomes of the people served by the organization.

Successful organizations, whether formal or informal, define themselves as open systems that operate within larger community systems and social networks, and facilitate support networks for people with ID-DD and their families. These larger systems are considered as resources for the organization, and the organization plans for and uses the resources of community, social networks, and support networks in facilitating personal outcomes.

Thinking of the organization as part of a community system or resource network creates many more potential opportunities and supportive resources for people striving to attain their personal outcomes. Community sectors in the areas of health, housing, employment, education, transportation, leisure, and social capital offer potential resources for facilitating personal outcomes.

Leadership

As shown in Figure 4.3, management for QOL outcomes requires leadership in terms of (a) organizational vision, values, and expectations regarding people with disabilities, and (b) culture, behavior, and performance that provides the supports to address expectations. Let's look at this required leadership as it relates to three concepts: (a) organizational dynamics, (b) leadership themes, and (c) investment in direct-support professional leadership.

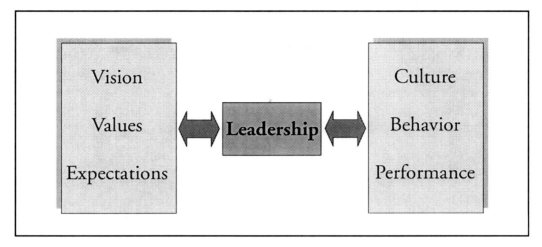

Figure 4.3. Function of quality leadership in a service-based organization.

Organizational Dynamics

Organizations are dynamic, not static. To help explain this, Bolman and Deal (2003) have provided a model based on four categorical frames of organizational dynamics: (a) the rational and structural, (b) the human resource, (c) the political, and (d) the symbolic. Each framework offers a unique analysis of goal setting, resource allocation, and power distribution. People with ID-DD, as the end users, must direct the organization. With that statement in mind, let's consider organizational leadership questions applicable in each of the four frames.

Rational and Structural

Within this framework, decisions are made in a logical and analytical manner. The strongest argument, the most persuasive analysis, or the clearest statement leads to organizational goals and priorities. Boyle (2001) notes that what we count, and how well we count, shape the definition of what's important, and that the most well-reasoned and convincing arguments often establish goals. Questions to consider: How do organizations frame issues, describe options, and facilitate input to enable people with disabilities to exercise real leadership? Do people with ID-DD have the resources and supports to make their arguments and support their positions in organizational debates and decision making?

Human Resource

Within this framework, decisions are made to promote harmony and consensus. The least disruptive decisions lead to organizational goals. Questions to consider: In resolving conflict and reaching consensus within organizations, do the interests of people with ID-DD match those of other stakeholders? Or do organizations resolve conflict and reach consensus with only nominal recognition of individuals served?

Political or Power Based

Within this framework, decisions are made by those who possess the power and influence. Conflicts over goals are decided by those with power. Questions to consider: Do people with ID-DD hold the political power to set or influence the goals and mission of the organization? If ultimate goals and mission reflect self-interest, do people with disabilities wield enough organizational influence? Are they even at the table when the key decisions are made?

Symbolic

Within this framework, decisions are made in regard to the status, prestige, and value of the symbols most important to the organization. Individuals and groups aligned with the most important status and symbols set the goals. Questions to consider: Do people with ID-DD have access to powerful and positive symbols? What values, images, and symbolism do people with disabilities convey within the organization and community? Do others associate people with ID-DD with powerful and positive symbols?

Bolman and Deal (2003) note that organizational dynamics often fall into one of the above categorical frames. But organizations can also exhibit elements from several frames. In some instances, organizational behavior can be explained by all four frames. Our concern here is not to identify frames most commonly exhibited by organizations providing services and supports to people with ID-DD; rather, readers should understand that no matter what frame best explains organizational behavior, organizations need to examine, understand, and strengthen the leadership and goal-setting capacity of people with disabilities in whatever frame the organization operates.

Leadership Themes

As shown in Figure 4.3, one aspect of leadership is the management of the organization's performance in facilitating people's outcomes. There is an abundance of research literature on leadership within human services and nonprofit organizations. We note several leadership themes that are particularly relevant in facilitating enhanced QOL outcomes for people with ID-DD.

Servant Leadership

In this model organizational leaders support other people within the organization in their efforts. This is an inverted pyramid model where the leaders are obligated to other organizational members and stakeholders (Greenleaf, 1991).

Participant Action Research

There are two parts to this theme (French & Bell, 1998). The first stresses the role of the participant. Leaders from throughout the organization are the participants in a continuous examination of quality of life. They are analyzing their own leadership and quality initiatives. The second involves action research, which stresses the importance of taking action and then learning from those actions. Organizational leaders learn by doing; they demonstrate a bias toward acting. They then examine the actions and the consequences resulting from the action. They open the doors inward and learn about people, how to facilitate outcomes, and how to improve supports. This participant action research model builds on organizational strengths and capacity. It links strengths and resources with the process of organizational learning and quality improvement and is grounded in the realities of people's lives.

This model of action research suggests that leaders gather enough information to make reasonable decisions, but the decision is then tested and analyzed by the results. Action research is an alternative to the traditional planning model that attempts to plan and analyze prior to acting. Action research with an imperative to "change lives now" suggests that organizations take prudent action, learn from their actions, and engage in repeated cycles of action research.

Action-centered management and leadership skills of successful executives have been well documented in management literature (Isenberg, 1984; Kotter, 1982; Mintzberg, 1973; Vail, 1993; Zuboff, 1988). Wheatley (1994) summarized this need to learn from doing with the notation that "Knowing the steps ahead of time is not important; being willing to engage with the music and move freely onto the dance floor is what's key" (p. 143).

Community Leadership

Organizational leaders recognize that lives and quality of life flourish in the community. Organizations, by themselves, simply cannot offer the range of opportunities and life experiences available in the community. Leaders use organizations as bridges to the community, and the leaders indeed lead the organization into the community. Facilitating QOL outcomes requires leaders to position their organizations as high-status, visible, and leading civic organizations that enhance social capital for all their members.

Cultural Directors

Organizational leaders set and reinforce values, symbols, and priorities (i.e., organizational culture) by paying attention to particular aspects of organizational life. Effective leaders are focused. They pay attention to those aspects of organizational life that maximize QOL outcomes for people. They constantly (a) place people with ID-DD in the position to direct organizational priorities, direct their own supports, and direct feedback on and evaluation of organizational performance; (b) reinforce people for appropriate performance and behavior; (c) pay attention to data and information about QOL outcomes; and (d) communicate the centrality of personal outcomes to the organization's purpose and mission.

In summary, organizational leadership is essential in facilitating personal outcomes. The literature clearly identifies three relevant leadership themes: servant leadership, community leadership, and cultural directors. However, organizations also need to invest in direct-support professional leadership.

Investment in Direct-Support Professional Leadership

Direct-support professionals are directly responsible for delivering on the promise of basic assurances and fulfillment of personal outcomes made to service recipients. Direct-support professionals have the opportunity to continuously learn about people's outcomes and the particular (and often innovative) supports that will facilitate them. More important, direct-support professionals have the opportunity to facilitate outcomes that require personal understanding and a commitment to personal outcomes.

Over the past decade our experience and research has yielded new information on direct-support professionals. Our purpose in this section is not to summarize or synthesize that information (see, e.g., Larson, Lakin, & Hewitt, 2002). We do, however, point out key managerial approaches that encourage and assist direct-support professionals in defining their careers and work in terms of personal outcome attainment.

Recruitment and Hiring

Recruitment and hiring are based on the aptitude for and attitude toward facilitating personal outcomes. These personality traits are more important than skills and techniques, which can be addressed through training and education programs. The recruitment and hiring process brings together people receiving services and supports with their potential providers. Thus hiring decisions require input from people being supported.

Retention, Supervision, and Support

The key variable influencing retention and the quality of the supports is the support the professionals themselves receive. This support from middle management is highly personal. Mid-level managers participate in the learning, planning, and provision of supports related to outcomes. Mid-level managers interact regularly with direct-support professionals in the provision of those supports, giving ongoing feedback and encouragement.

Salary, Health Care, and Other Organizational Supports

Direct-support professionals generally belong to the occupational classification of low-wage workers. The information about low-wage workers suggests that salary, while low, remains important, because it directly impacts their ability to support themselves and their families. For this reason, health care is critical. So also are the other supports of daycare, transportation, housing, and education. Because low-wage workers generally have limited resources, their support systems are fragile. Breakdowns in one area of support place even greater demands on the other supports, and the fragile systems that direct-support professionals require for employment can become strained and eventually break. The values and principles that facilitate outcomes for people with ID-DD—self-directed goals and services, natural supports, appreciative inquiry, servant leadership—also enhance the development of successful employees.

Social Capital

The themes of personal outcomes and social capital can be powerful motivators for direct-support professionals. Three direct benefits result from increased social capital for direct-support professionals: (a) The physical, psychological, and emotional benefits of social capital accrue over time; (b) increased social capital for direct-support professionals increases and strengthens their own support network; accrued social capital creates alternative solutions and resources in times when their once fragile support networks might have broken; and (c) direct-support professionals are better able to facilitate opportunities for social capital for people with disabilities when they are connected and building their own network of relationships.

Potential for Knowledge Expansion

Direct-support professionals directly influence the rate of transfer of tacit to explicit knowledge. Within the organization they have a key role in the exchange of knowledge and information. By learning from doing, listening to stories, observing the creation of organizational myth and heroes, and facilitating outcomes, they have access to knowledge and information that is often not available to other employees. The direct-support professionals are then challenged to convey that tacit information within the organization and also to convert it into explicit knowledge for the organization.

This potential for knowledge expansion on the part of direct-support professionals creates several challenges for organizational management. On the one hand, organizations need to recognize and respect the value of tacit knowledge. They must create a place and opportunity for the exchange of this tacit knowledge. On the other hand, they must promote the translation of the tacit knowledge into the explicit knowledge that can be codified, reproduced, and disseminated. They must invest in direct-support professionals, to both encourage and expand the tacit knowledge base as well as direct that tacit knowledge and understanding into formal organizational channels.

Summary

Managing for personal outcomes requires a foundation in the values and principles derived from self-determination, inclusion, social capital, and legal and human rights. However, values by themselves are not sufficient to bring about personal outcomes for people with ID-DD. Managing for personal outcomes requires skill and ability.

The skills, abilities, and experiences related to leadership, organizational coordination, negotiation and conflict resolution, and an understanding of organizational design and behavior make values and principles "come alive." Better interview methods, new formats and designs for self-directed services and supports, dissemination of model programs, and promising practices will make a difference only if they are coupled with successful implementation and management.

The most powerful values and principles are derived from the universal themes of social justice, human rights, social inclusion, and economic opportunity. The successful application and implementation of these universal themes deserve no less than the very best from our leadership in the field. To that end, this chapter has outlined a new way to think about managerial strategies and the importance of opening the door inward. Specifically, we have suggested that for personal outcomes to be met, organizations need to transition to more individualized, dispersed support systems, and thereby address five critical factors that make a personal outcome system work: strategy, execution, culture, structure, and leadership. The material presented in this chapter builds on what we know about social capital, organizational processes that facilitate personal outcomes, leadership models and organizational culture, human resource development strategies, the community as a resource, and how to nurture and sustain healthy organizations.

Personal outcomes and their measurement are basic to the organizational change process. The following chapter discusses one approach—that of the Council on Quality and Leadership—to measuring personal outcomes within the context of innovation and an integrated management system.

CHAPTER 5

Personal Outcome Measures: Values and Metrics for an Integrated Management System

Introduction and Overview

In the past quarter century, self-advocates and their families, service and support providers, and the federal, state, and local governments have altered historical patterns of disability services. Litigation, legislation, and increased public sector funding have fueled this social transformation. Throughout this period of change, our framework for assessing quality has lagged behind the changing patterns of service and support provision, self-determination, and choice. As services and supports have changed, our definitions and expectations for quality have grown. But as Jaskulski (1991) noted, these changes have resulted in discontinuities and overlaps. New concepts never totally replace older traditions. Instead, innovation in human services coexists and evolves with traditional practices, which results in the paradox of innovation.

The Paradox of Innovation

Organizations supporting people with intellectual and developmental disabilities (ID-DD) confront a dilemma. In pursuing innovation and creative alternatives, organizations often find a lack of clear procedural guidelines and criteria for determining quality of the supports they procure or provide. What's more, existing regulations, guidelines, and criteria for determining quality are often outdated. The paradox is that the current definitions and measurement of quality are often grounded in priorities and practices from the past century, and the new priorities and practices have not yet generated a consensus that will satisfy all stakeholders. The result is that innovation and creativity coexist with older, but accepted, practices and definitions of quality.

This paradox confronts human service organizations for several reasons. First, many human service organizations are not-for-profit and thus lack a bottom-line focus that drives change and innovation in the business sector. Second, legislation, regulation, and public oversight are slow to change. Public sector change depends on a time-consuming evolution in consensus. Third, human service organizational performance is measured and evaluated by legacy data and information systems. As a result, even the most innovative organizations often rely on traditional data- and quality-measurement systems.

Minimizing the Paradox

Organizations cannot escape this paradox. Indeed, as discussed in the preceding chapter, organizations need leadership that can successfully balance current realities with emerging innovation and thereby manage this paradox. In addition, organizations require an integrated, value-based quality system, such as that shown in Figure 5.1. Such a system is also comprehensive, integrated, and dynamic.

Value Based

Values will assign meanings to the design, definition, and measurement of factors of quality. Values related to person-directed choice, planning, and self-determination will ensure that quality factors reflect a concern and respect for people receiving services and supports.

Comprehensive

The integrated quality system includes *quality assurance* factors that address basic

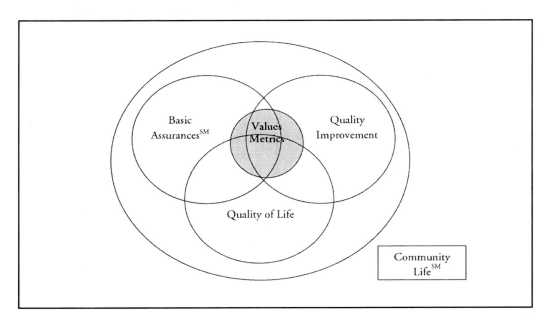

Figure 5.1. Integrated quality system for an organization providing disability services.

Note. Copyright 2005 by the Council on Quality and Leadership. Reprinted with permission.

assurances in health, safety, and human security as well as financial, legal, and management compliance requirements. The system also addresses organizational *quality improvement* and includes factors related to efficiency and effectiveness. A comprehensive quality system also emphasizes personal *quality of life* (QOL) outcomes, including factors related to choice, self-determination, and well-being.

Integrated

Quality system factors are integrated so that organizations can incorporate these factors into a quality-management system where values and metrics coincide. The quality system begins with person-directed values and uses a single set of person-directed metrics to assess the factors of quality assurance, quality improvement, and quality of life.

Dynamic

The quality system is also dynamic and supports (a) information and data analysis; (b) changes in policy, procedure, and practice; and (c) organizational action strategies designed to improve quality performance. The data and information in a quality-management system have multiple applications. The same data and information can be used (a) for person-directed planning; (b) to address basic assurances in health, safety, and human security; (c) to benchmark individual QOL outcomes and organizational-supports performance against other organizations and systems; and (d) to change organizational and community supports to enhance quality of life.

Chapter Focus and Definitions

This chapter focuses on the Personal QOL Outcome Measures developed by the Council on Quality and Leadership (CQL). The *Personal Outcome Measures* (CQL, 1997, 2000d, 2005b)[1] are composed of 25 quality indicators (i.e., measures) reflecting five QOL domains: identity, autonomy, affiliation, attainment, safeguards, rights, and health and wellness. The measures are widely used (as described later in this chapter) for several reasons. First, the *Personal Outcome Measures* offer an integrated quality-management system for organizations, networks of organizations, and systems of service. Second, the values, methods, content, development, and application processes for these measures provide suggestions for organizations developing their own integrated quality-management systems. Third, since 1971 CQL has designed and developed measures and standards for quality in the field of ID-DD. CQL's definitions, measures, and organizational applications for quality have influenced and directed state and federal court decisions, national and state legislation, and regulation and organizational practice. With representation from leading national advocacy, provider, and professional organizations, CQL includes and addresses a broad constituency in the field of ID-DD (Gardner, 2002; Gardner & Nudler, 1999; Hemp

---

[1] All subsequent mentions of the measures refer to this reference citation.

& Braddock, 1990).

The following definitions guide our discussion through this chapter:

• *Quality assurance:* Quality oversight that addresses a support or service provider's demonstrated ability to guarantee basic assurances in the areas of health, safety, and continuity.

• *Quality improvement:* Individual, organizational, or systems capacity to improve performance and accountability through systematically collecting and analyzing data and information and implementing action strategies based on the analysis.

• *Quality of life:* A focus on the personal outcomes as defined by each person receiving services and supports. Quality assurance and quality-improvement initiatives enhance the quality of life for people.

CQL and the Design for Change

CQL is an international quality design, measurement, and performance improvement organization. CQL's quality initiatives are directed to people with ID-DD and people with mental illness and the people, organizations, and systems that support them.

CQL originated in the late 1960s as a national accreditation organization. The need for accreditation standards arose from abuses and harsh custodial care in residential institutions. During the early 1970s, CQL issued the first accreditation standards for organizations serving people with intellectual disabilities. Over the next 20 years, standards of the Accreditation Council on Services for People With Mental Retardation and Other Developmental Disabilities were incorporated into the Intermediate Care Facility Program for the Mentally Retarded (ICF-MR) regulations, the *Wyatt v. Stickney* (2000) decision, and state licensing requirements (Gardner, 2002; Gardner & Nudler, 1999; Hemp & Braddock, 1990).

CQL initiated a review of its standards in 1990 (Accreditation Council on Services for People With Disabilities, 1993). Despite the comprehensiveness of its 810 accreditation standards, the process-driven procedural requirements were failing to promote quality in services. In response to this situation, CQL's board of directors began to develop the personal outcome measures in 1991. The new quality measures had four design requirements: (a) concise; (b) generic (applying to a wide range of people receiving diverse services and supports); (c) person, not program, focused; and (d) integrated in regard to management applications. These requirements posed two significant challenges. The first was to develop a valid and reliable set of outcomes, indicators, and performance measures that were not prescriptive. Focus groups of people with disabilities identified generic outcomes that people felt were most important in their own lives: friends, health, money, work, family, and place to live. CQL then developed a rigorous and reliable methodology for determining whether or not the outcome, as defined by the person, was present or not in that person's life.

Five application requirements also guided the work.

1. Individual measurement items would have a personal meaning and application for each individual. The measures could be used in, or support, various forms of person-directed planning.

2. In addition to providing information about individuals, the outcome data could be aggregated across settings, organizations, and systems.

3. When organizations determined the presence or lack of outcomes, they could at the same time identify supports that, if provided, would or probably would facilitate the outcome. The organizations could then analyze the supports in terms of values and mission, organizational structure, personnel, and budget.

4. Organizational performance improvement could be monitored by personal outcome and supports data.

5. Organizations could define and measure basic assurances in the areas of health, safety, freedom from abuse and neglect, and human security using the personal outcomes as well as applicable supports and the policies and procedures that define those supports.

Values and Principles of Personal Outcome Measures

The content and face validity of the *Personal Outcome Measures* results from direct, in-person participation by people with disabilities and/or mental illness and their families and supporters in the design and development process. We used individual and focus-group input for the initial design of the personal outcomes. Subsequent revisions have also incorporated individual interviews and focus-group feedback. Both the content of the *Personal Outcome Measures* and the interview and information collection methodology are grounded in the theory and practice of self-directed decision making (Gardner & Carran, 2005; Gardner, Nudler, & Chapman, 1997). The logic of the *Personal Outcome Measures* is contained in the following: (a) people define their own outcomes; (b) the process of identifying and defining outcomes is experiential; people experience a range of options from which to make choices; and (c) organizations provide the supports to facilitate those outcomes identified and defined by the individual. Reflective of this logic are the following six values and principles: (a) dimensions of choice, (b) discovering preferences, (c) organizational responsibility, (d) individuality, (e) objective measurement of person-centered quality of life measures, and (f) the individualization of organizational process.

Dimensions of Choice

For individuals to make meaningful choices and decisions, the process must include three dimensions.

Experiential Context for Choice

People need concrete life experiences related to possible choices. The support organization has the responsibility to provide the person with training, counseling, and opportunities to experience and try the options involved in making choices. In some cases, people with more significant disabilities may require additional supports, experiences, and options from which to choose to make outcomes possible and relevant.

Social Context for Choice

Social support networks assist people in making choices. Most people seek advice from family, friends, and peers when faced with significant or difficult choices. They seldom make hard decisions by themselves. People need regular access to groups of trusted peers, friends, and family to share feelings and information and to seek support and counsel.

Creative Context for Choice

Choices and decisions seldom consist of an either-or situation. Instead, most people attempt to find creative alternatives to a forced choice between Choice A and Choice B. This search for creative compromise between apparent givens contributes to personal esteem and satisfaction. The support organization has a responsibility to assist people in identifying creative alternatives that meet their individual needs and expectations, yet fit with obtainable or available resources. This search for creative alternatives is greatly enhanced when organizations search beyond the boundaries of their own supports and programs. Creative alternatives most often derive from social networks and other community connections.

Discovering Preferences

Support organizations often find it difficult to discover or understand people's personal outcomes. In these situations, the measures retain their importance, but the discovery mode changes. Support organizations make the transition from communicating about choice to discovering preferences. Direct-support professionals, clinicians, families, and friends share information about the individual's preferences. This discovery of preferences takes place daily; in many instances it results from accumulated informal or tacit information gathered during daily interactions. In some instances, a direct-support professional may need assistance in translating the informal information of feelings, observations, or "knowing" into personal outcome statements of preferences. We know from experience that all people have preferences—the people they want around them, the side of their bodies they prefer to sleep on, or the nourishment they need.

The same dimensions of choice cited earlier apply to the discovery of preferences. People are given a range of experiences and opportunities. They are also provided with ongoing support while learning from experience and indicating preferences. Finally, support providers, families, and friends, as creatively as possible, offer an array of experiences that may extend beyond the scope of the support organization itself. In some cases this discovery period may take months; a commitment to detect preferences requires not only creativity, but also patience, and a willingness to start over and try again.

Organizational Responsibility

These conditions for making choices or discovering preferences—experiencing a range of choices, offering social support in making choices, and working creatively to define choices—must be present before an outcome is considered met. Without these dimensions, people cannot have real choice in, for example, where to work, where and with whom to live, or whom to call "friend." Only real choice can define the presence of an outcome.

Individuality

The *Personal Outcome Measures* are self-defined and described. This is true despite a comprehensive development process involving focus groups meetings with people with ID-DD, field testing over 4 years, and revisions based on analysis of our national database (CQL, 2005f). People nevertheless continue to identify their own definitions for each of the outcome categories. For example, each person will assign an individual meaning to items such as "people are respected" and "people participate in the life of the community." What constitutes respect is, after all, different for us all.

Thus the 25 Personal Outcome Measures do not contain a normative or scaled measure of their outcomes. Each person is a unique sample of one. No norm or standardized definition exists that can have meaning for different people. That is why it is essential that individuals have their own unique definitions for each of the outcome measures.

Objective Measurement of Person-Centered Quality of Life Measures

Organizations determine the presence or absence of outcomes based on information and data gathered during on-site, in-person interactions with respondents, surrogates, and other information sources. Interviewers follow a decision tree matrix in these interactions. In this way, organizations can gain and analyze information from both a structured and open-ended interview process within a framework of decision guides and questions specific to each of the 25 outcome measures.

Thus the outcomes are not self-reported, nor do they measure personal opinion (of either the respondent, surrogate, other information source, or interviewer) or report respondent satisfaction for each of the outcome questions. In developing the *Personal Outcome Measures*, we recognized the difficulty and complexity of obtaining reliable and valid information from some people with significant disabilities and the people who support them. We attempted to minimize these challenges by requiring multiple decision sources, a decision tree matrix model, and repeated questioning for several hours spread over different times with multiple respondents in different settings.

Individualizing the Organization's Process

Using the *Personal Outcome Measures* results in an organization's identifying the personal meaning of the outcomes for each individual. This focus on personal outcomes forms the basis for the organization's process of person-directed planning. In addition, each of the personal outcome measures contains a series of individualized support questions that follow from the interviewee's answer to the outcome question. The support questions determine (a) whether individual supports currently facilitate that outcome, or (b) in cases where an outcome is not present, whether identified supports would facilitate that outcome. These supports are not programs or standardized processes. Rather, they are the individualized actions that organizations take to facilitate the outcome as defined by the person.

This individual approach shifts organizational strategy and design from programs to people. Instead of maintaining uniform organizational processes by program, organizations must now individualize processes to facilitate personally defined outcomes. This change has two consequences. The first is that human services, like the commercial manufacturing sector, are replacing uniform mass production (through programs) with individualized design. The second implication is more subtle, though profound. No one else can identify or define the individualized process until the person has defined his or her meaning of the outcome.

This individualization of process reverses the traditional total quality management and continuous quality improvement approach. Because the ends (the individualized meaning of the outcome) differ, the processes that support people to achieve those outcomes will also differ. Human service organizations, after all, are not interested in constructing the kind of uniform product (e.g., a toaster) that results from a continuous and consistent process. If all people receiving services and supports defined all personal outcome measures in the same manner, and if all these people learned and interacted with other people in the same way, the process might be standardized. However, because different people define their outcomes distinctively, the process to facilitate the outcome will vary.

Thus we can draw a significant conclusion for QOL measurement. It is not feasible to measure an organization's individualized supports-planning processes without first identifying the outcomes around which the process is designed.

CQL Research, Development, and Continued Refinement

During the continued development of the *Personal Outcome Measures*, CQL has revisited their validity, reliability, and application (Gardner & Carran, 2005; Gardner, Carran, & Nudler, 2001; Gardner & Nudler, 1999; Gardner, Nudler, & Chapman, 1997). The methodology for applying the measures has been widely disseminated (CQL, 2000a–2000g). We have described the methodology for gathering information from people who do not communicate or who use nontraditional communication methods (CQL, 2000a, 2000b). CQL's design, development, and continued refinement of the Personal Outcome Measures address issues of reliability, consistency, and usable analysis. These issues are important for any organization or system that develops a quality-management system.

The Reliability of Data

CQL (2005f) includes in its national database only personal outcome data collected by certified personal outcome interviewers. All CQL staff and certified interviewers must achieve a .85 level of interrater reliability with senior "gold standard" CQL staff.

The Consistency of Data Collection

CQL (2005f) includes in its national database only personal outcome data collected by certified personal outcome interviewers during accreditation reviews. The accreditation review protocol identifies the processes and procedures for conducting interviews, collecting information, investigating and eliminating discrepancies, and making scoring decisions for each of the personal outcomes for each person interviewed. Thus interviews conducted by certified interviewers during self-assessment workshops, values alignment exercises, or basic certifications are not entered into the national database.

The Analysis of Data

CQL continually refines its *Personal Outcome Measures* based on an analysis of data. Any changes have been guided by our analysis of each item's functionality and utility in discriminating quality and by the factor analysis of the set of outcomes. In addition, the analysis of the data has changed the way we manage the organization, the quality strategies that we offer to customers, and the way we think about quality for the future.

A National Personal Outcome Measures Database

The values and principles of the *Personal Outcome Measures* provide the foundation for a valid and reliable measurement system that integrates requirements for quality assurance, quality improvement, and QOL attainment. Self-advocates, families and supporters, organizations, and systems can use the *Personal Outcome Measures* to evaluate their own performance, accomplishments over time, and remaining challenges and gaps in quality. In addition, the national *Personal Outcome Measures* database (CQL, 2005f) enables individuals, services, organizations, and systems to compare their quality performance with similar or different efforts throughout the United States. Although the national database uses the entire sample of personal outcome measures interviews, users can select variables for application in their own quality improvement and benchmarking activity.

A National Snapshot

The national database (CQL, 2005f) currently contains *Personal Outcome Measures* data and information on more than 5,000 individuals who participated in personal outcome interviews during accreditation reviews in more than 600 organizations in the period 1992–2004. A summary of the data on outcomes and organizational supports in place for the sample population appears in Table 5.1. The outcomes column indicates the percentage of people in the national sample for whom the outcome is present. The supports column shows the percentage with which specific supports are (a) present and facilitate attainment of the outcome, or (b) in place and expected to result in the outcome. The organizational supports data indicates an organization's success in individualizing its resources and processes to address personal outcomes. These data allow an organization to assess its accountability and accomplishments in supporting people to achieve their defined personal outcomes.

TABLE 5.1

Summary of Data on Personal Measurement Outcomes and Organizational Supports Collected Nationwide During Accreditation Reviews

Personal Measurement Outcomes	% of Outcomes Present	% of Supports Present
Domain: Identity		
1. People choose personal goals.	46.1	46.6
2. People choose where and with whom to live.	44.3	55.2
3. People choose where they work.	38.3	49.1
4. People have intimate relationships.	72.4	67.4
5. People are satisfied with services.	87.3	81.2
6. People are satisfied with their personal life.	85.5	85.6
Domain: Autonomy		
7. People choose their daily routines.	84.6	84.1
8. People have time, space, and opportunity for privacy.	90.1	91.6
9. People decide when to share personal information.	79.2	69.1
10. People use their environments.	76.7	79.0
Domain: Affiliation		
11. People live in integrated environments.	34.8	41.7
12. People participate in the life of the community.	74.0	80.6
13. People interact with other members of the community.	71.1	73.1
14. People perform different social roles.	31.6	31.3
15. People have friends.	57.8	59.0
16. People are respected.	77.1	80.2

(table continues)

Table 5.1 *(continued)*

Personal Measurement Outcomes	% of Outcomes Present	% of Supports Present
Domain: Attainment		
17. People choose services.	45.7	47.4
18. People realize personal goals.	82.6	82.0
Domain: Safeguards		
19. People remain connected to natural support networks.	64.4	77.6
20. People are safe.	86.9	81.7
Domain: Rights		
21. People exercise rights.	42.9	39.6
22. People are treated fairly.	50.4	50.1
Domain: Health and Wellness		
23. People have the best possible health.	73.5	72.8
24. People are free from abuse and neglect.	86.2	89.8
25. People experience continuity and security.	81.8	78.4

Note. $N = 5,542$. 2005 statistics are based on data collected during accreditation reviews in more than 600 organizations from 1992–2004 by the Council on Quality and Leadership. *National Database, 2005.* Accessible online at: www.cfl.org.

Benchmarking and Comparisons

A valid and reliable national database enables organizations, networks, and systems to benchmark their own quality management and organizational performance improvement efforts in relation to those of similar service types, organizations, and systems throughout the country. For example, Table 5.2 illustrates how organizations can benchmark their own performance against national performance on the Personal Outcome Measures and individualized supports.

When analyzing this outcome and support data, organizations also identify the type and frequency of the support producing or leading to the outcome. This descriptive and qualitative information enables organizations to link QOL measures with specific, individualized supports for each of the 25 Personal Outcome Measures. In addition, organizations can benchmark their performance for both outcomes and supports by characteristics of people supported, such as age or disability, type of residential supports (e.g., independent living, supported living, supervised living, natural or foster family), source of funding (e.g., state and/or federal support or resource), or size and location of organization.

	TABLE 5.2					
	Sample Benchmarking and Comparison Data for Alpha, Inc.					
	National[a]		Alpha, Inc.		Differences	
Personal Measurement Outcomes	% of Outcomes Present	% of Supports Present	% of Outcomes Present	% of Supports Present	% of Outcomes Present	% of Supports Present
1. Choose personal goals	46.10	46.60	52.63	41.58	6.5	-5.0
2. Choose where and with whom to live	44.30	55.20	31.58	46.84	-12.7	-8.4
3. Choose where they work	38.30	49.10	34.41	36.84	-3.9	-12.3
4. Have intimate relationships	72.40	67.40	70.60	68.42	-1.8	1.0
5. Are satisfied with services	87.30	81.20	73.68	64.42	-13.6	-16.8
6. Are satisfied with their personal life	85.50	85.60	83.49	84.21	-2.0	-1.4
7. Choose their daily routines	84.60	84.10	84.21	78.42	-0.4	-5.7
8. Have time, space, and opportunity for privacy	90.10	91.60	86.30	88.95	-3.8	-2.6
9. Decide when to share personal information	79.20	69.10	73.68	84.21	-5.5	15.1
10. Use their environments	76.70	79.00	78.95	78.95	2.2	-0.1
11. Live in integrated environments	34.80	41.70	31.58	42.11	-3.2	0.4
12. Participate in the life of the community	74.00	80.60	72.63	73.16	-1.4	-7.4
13. Interact with other members of the community	71.10	73.10	84.21	78.95	13.1	5.8
14. Perform different social roles	31.60	31.30	21.05	21.05	-10.5	-10.2

(table continues)

TABLE 5.2 *(continued)*

Personal Measurement Outcomes	National[a]		Alpha, Inc.		Differences	
	% of Outcomes Present	% of Supports Present	% of Outcomes Present	% of Supports Present	% of Outcomes Present	% of Supports Present
15. Have friends	57.80	59.00	57.89	66.84	0.1	7.8
16. Are respected	77.10	80.20	89.47	88.95	12.4	8.8
17. Choose services	45.70	47.40	57.89	57.89	12.2	10.5
18. Realize personal goals	82.60	82.00	63.16	57.89	-19.4	-24.1
19. Remain connected to natural support networks	64.40	77.60	52.63	52.63	-11.8	-25.0
20. Are safe	86.90	81.70	89.47	89.47	2.6	7.8
21. Exercise rights	42.90	39.60	73.68	68.42	30.8	28.8
22. Are treated fairly	50.40	50.10	73.68	78.95	23.3	28.8
23. Have the best possible health	73.50	72.80	84.21	73.16	10.7	0.4
24. Are free from abuse and neglect	86.20	89.80	89.47	89.47	3.3	-0.3
25. Experience continuity and security	81.80	78.40	84.21	83.16	2.4	4.8

[a]*N = 5,542*. 2005 statistics are based on data collected during accreditation reviews in more than 600 organizations from 1992–2004 by the Council on Quality and Leadership. *National Database, 2005*. Accessible online at: www.cfl.org.

Data, Information, and Decision Making

Organizations and systems of supports can use the outcome and support data to make decisions about types of services and supports, public policy and funding priorities, expectations for their own quality-management systems, and the relationship between choice and basic assurances and personal wellness.

Services and Supports

The national database and databases maintained by organizations and systems will provide information on the relationship between outcomes and supports and the size and types of supports that influence attaining personal outcome measures. Organizations can use the national as well as their own *Personal Outcome Measures* databases to decide how to allocate resources and structure support services. For example, small and moderately sized organizations serving 26 to 200 individuals have a higher percentage of outcomes compared to very small (< 25) or very large (> 200) organizations. We also know that (a) size of organization may be more critical to people with more severe disabilities, and (b) people with disabilities, regardless of kind of disability, achieve more outcomes in supported living settings than in supervised settings (Gardner & Carran, 2005).

Policy and Funding Priorities
In a similar manner, an analysis of the CQL national database by type of funding (HCBS waiver or ICF-MR) indicates that regardless of disability, the lowest percentage of outcomes were present for ICF-MRs. For individuals with severe or profound mental retardation, the percentage of outcomes in HCBS-funded services were significantly higher than in ICF-MRs. Individual organizations, networks, and public systems of support can use similar databases to answer questions of how to best direct funding to promote the optimal quality of life for people (Gardner & Carran, 2005).

Relationship Among Variables
Organizations can ask and answer questions about the impact of choosing where to live or where to work on other outcomes, such as health, safety, and freedom from abuse and neglect. The national database can provide analysis of the impact of community affiliation (e.g., social roles, friendships, and participation in the life of the community) on outcomes related to basic assurances and choice. From an analysis of our data (Gardner & Carran, 2005), we know that (a) choice did not affect the outcome of the "people are safe" indicator, but that choice does have a modest positive relationship with "people are free from abuse and neglect"; and (b) when three choice outcomes—services, work, and residence—were present, an individual was three times more likely to have the outcome of social roles also present.

Quality-Management Systems Measurement: What's the Question?
The personal outcome databases maintained by organizations and systems can also address issues related to quality of services and quality of life. For example, we can analyze the difference between outcomes that predict organizational accreditation and outcomes that predict quality of life (Gardner & Carran, 2005).

Table 5.3 identifies the top five predictors of accreditation. These predictors were generally outcomes directly related to organizational processes and the values originating from within the organization's existing services. These outcomes are generally facilitated by services and supports originating from within the organization's existing programs. Table 5.3 also identifies the top five predictors for achieving the largest number of personal outcomes. Only one of these outcomes, "people are respected," is among the best predictors of accreditation. The other four are not (i.e., "people choose where and with whom to live"; "people choose where they work"; "people interact with other members of the community"; and "people exercise rights").

TABLE 5.3

Predictions of Quality of Life and Accreditation Outcomes

Quality of Life

1. Choose where and with whom they live (Outcome 2)

2. Exercise rights (Outcome 21)

3. Interact with members of the community (Outcome 13)

4. Are respected (Outcome 16)

5. Choose where they work (Outcome 3)

Accreditation

1. Are treated fairly (Outcome 22)

2. Realize personal goals (Outcome 18)

3. Are respected (Outcome 16)

4. Choose personal goals (Outcome 1)

5. Participate in the life of the community (Outcome 12)

Table 5.4 identifies the top five predictors of achieving the largest number of outcomes for different sectors of people. These analyses are particularly important for organizational resource planning. Facilitating personal outcomes begins with the allocation of resources for support services. Organizations can then use data to answer two questions: (a) Have we initiated the supports that will facilitate intended outcomes? and (b) Are we allocating resources and providing supports that are not linked to people's personal outcomes?

Analysis and interpretation of an organization's personal measurement outcome data indicate that organizations have greater difficulty responding to personal outcomes that involve options beyond those offered by the organization itself. Facilitating each person's definition of community living, work, and social interaction remains a significant challenge.

Applications and Quality Strategies

Organizations incorporate the *Personal Outcome Measures* and their various applications in their quality-improvement efforts through (a) coevaluation efforts with the CQL, or (b) individual use (recognizing copyright protections). Because the applications and measurement are based on the same personal outcome factors, indicators, and organizational supports, organizations can integrate their quality initiatives into a

TABLE 5.4

Outcomes That Predict Achieving the Largest Number of Personal Outcomes

By All People	By People With More Severe Intellectual Disability	By People With Intellectual Disability	By People With Mental Illness
Choose where and with whom they live (Outcome 2)	Interact with other members of the community (Outcome 13)	Choose where and with whom they live (Outcome 2)	Are afforded due process (Outcome 22)
Exercise rights (Outcome 21)	Are afforded due process (Outcome 22)	Exercise rights (Outcome 21)	Interact with other members of the community (Outcome 13)
Interact with other members of the community (Outcome 13)	Have intimate relationships (Outcome 4)	Are respected (Outcome 16)	Choose where and with whom they live (Outcome 2)
Are respected (Outcome 16)	Choose their daily routines (Outcome 7)	Choose where they work (Outcome 3)	Satisfied with personal life (Outcome 6)
Choose where they work (Outcome 3)	Choose personal goals (Outcome 1)	Interact with other members of the community (Outcome 13)	Choose where they work (Outcome 3)

single quality-management system. The *Personal Outcome Measures* and their applications will support seven broad quality-improvement strategies within organizations and systems: (a) organizational or systems values alignment; (b) person-centered planning; (c) measuring quality of life with personal outcome measures; (e) certification in basic assurances of health, safety, and human security; (f) design and measurement for organizational performance improvement; and (g) accreditation.

Organizational or Systems Values Alignment

Organizations frequently begin an organizational assessment or performance review with an analysis of their mission statements and values. Organizations attempt to include in their values statements and missions the contemporary terms associated with best and promising practice. A values alignment enables an organization to probe deeper into the organization and determine if (a) all members of the organization including people served, their families, board members, senior management staff, and direct-support personnel agree upon and share the same values; (b) the values serve as a guide for the organization in setting its vision and mission; and (c) the organization has established specific plans and staff and volunteer responsibilities for realizing these values.

The values audit helps organizations examine current values and practices and determine if they are consistent with the values set forth in the *Personal Outcome Measures*. Values alignment is based on data and information gathered during interviews with people receiving supports, families, organizations, community sectors, and public officials. The resulting data on attainment of personal outcomes and the presence of individual supports can be compared with the information in the national or the organization's own *Personal Outcome Measures* database. Organizations also have the option of not benchmarking the data and asking focus groups of people with ID-DD, their families, and supporters for their interpretation of the data. In addition, organizations and systems can compare focus group results from different groups of people (e.g., direct-support professionals, community volunteers, and people with disabilities).

The values alignment is designed as an organizational self-assessment. Because of its values orientation, organizations will find gaps between their values (i.e., what ought to be) and the current realities (i.e., what is). Strong values and high expectations make the gaps between values and actions more pronounced. The purpose of the values alignment is to identify the gaps and ensure that the organization puts real strategies in place to overcome them. Our values must lead to practice. When practice approaches values attainment, organizations redefine values as leading-edge indicators.

Person-Centered Planning

Person-centered planning emerged in the 1990s as an alternative to individual program plans and individual habilitation planning (Newton & Horner, 2004). Although the formats and styles of the various planning modalities may differ, the central point of the person-directed planning model is that (a) the person, and those people closest to the person, identify QOL outcomes most important to them; (b) the person, together with supporters, identifies strategies to achieve those identified outcomes; and (c) neither the QOL outcomes nor the strategies to achieve them are limited to organizational services or supports. In contrast, people are encouraged to consider a range of desired future outcomes and implementation strategies that may require resources, services, and supports beyond the boundaries of any one organization.

Organizations use information gathered during *Personal Outcome Measures* interviews to develop the person-centered plan. From this perspective, the *Personal Outcome Measures* interview or discovery process becomes data and information gathering for the person-centered planning process. In addition, the *Personal Outcome Measures* provide a primary source of information about individuals, their QOL outcomes, and the presence or absence of those outcomes in the person's life. The measures also identify the resources and supports that are, or will, facilitate QOL outcomes.

To promote person-centered planning and self-determination by self-advocates, CQL has developed personal planning workbooks for people with ID-DD and for people with mental illness (CQL, 2001, 2002). (From a multiple regression analysis of its national database [2005f], CQL identified the eight personal outcomes that best predicted achieving a maximum number of outcomes.) Although the items are different for both groups, the workbook format is similar. For each of the eight personal outcomes, the workbook provides a set of questions to help individuals determine both their own definitions of the outcome and the importance of that outcome in their lives at that moment. People use the workbook to identify a set of goals or actions that will guide them toward achieving their important outcomes and a list of supports they will need along the way.

Measuring Quality of Life With Personal Outcome Measures
The content and application methodology of the *Personal Outcome Measures* offers organizations and service systems a valid, uniform, and reliable system for (a) identifying QOL outcomes as defined and described by each person for each of the 25 indicators, (b) determining the presence or absence of those outcomes in each person's life, and (c) identifying the supports that are facilitating or will facilitate the outcome.

Some organizations and systems collect this QOL outcome and support information for their person-centered planning process. Others do so as part of their quality monitoring and improvement system. Still others need data to get accreditation with CQL, the Commission on Accreditation of Rehabilitation Facilities, or the Joint Commission on Accreditation of Health Care Organizations. Finally, organizations gather this information in an effort to remain consistent with the federal Centers on Medicare and Medicaid Services Quality Framework and to demonstrate "evidence" for the HCBS waiver submission and review process (see chap. 6). Some states, such as Florida, Wisconsin, New Jersey, and South Carolina, have included the *Personal Outcome Measures* as part of their quality plan for the HCBS waiver.

Basic Assurances Review
Basic assurances are essential, fundamental, and nonnegotiable requirements for all service and support providers. They demonstrate successful operations in the areas of

health, safety, and human security. These assurances must be based on absolute minimum uniform requirements. When we discuss personal quality of life, responsive services, or community life, we expect to find differences that reflect diversity among communities, organizations, and groups of people. We can discuss different levels of quality service in restaurants, health clinics, or disability organizations. Unlike the values alignment where we expect a discrepancy between values and practice, however, for basic assurances there can be no discrepancy. Those organizations unable to meet the requirements of health, safety, and human security are not permitted to operate as public or private entities.

An organizational basic assurances review looks at the provision of fundamental safeguards from the *person's perspective*. While basic assurances require certain systems and policies and procedures, the effectiveness of the system or the policy is determined in practice, person by person. For example, our analysis of the *Personal Outcome Measures* database (CQL, 2005f; Gardner & Carran, 2005) indicates that the *Basic Assurances Personal Outcome Measures* are more likely to be present for people who have the most interaction with others outside the organization. Data from more than 5,000 personal-outcomes interviews show that people who remain connected to their natural support network are far less likely to be subject to abuse, are healthier, and are more likely to live in safe environments. Thus the metrics for the *Personal Outcome Measures* integrate outcomes and supports in the areas of basic assurances (CQL, 2005a) and social capital (CQL, 2005c).

CQL has developed a Basic Assurances Self-Assessment (CQL, 2005a) to assist organizations and systems in evaluating the organizational supports that promote individualized personal outcomes in the areas of health, safety, and human security. The self-assessment contains 10 factors, indicators, and specific probe questions for each indicator. The self-assessment can be used as a baseline tool to assess the status of an organization before any quality-management initiative. The factors and indicators can also measure the results of the quality-management initiative. The basic assurances outcomes are integrated with the indicators and metrics of organizational responsiveness. Basic assurances factors include: rights, protection, and promotion; dignity and respect; natural support networks; protection from abuse, neglect, mistreatment, and exploitation; best possible health; safe environments; staff resources and supports; positive services and supports; continuity and personal security; and a basic assurances system.

Organizational Performance or Quality Improvement

The development of the postindustrial, knowledge-based society in the middle and late 20th century challenged the foundations of industrial-era organizational management. Organizations, both business and nonprofit, developed new approaches to quality management and organizational performance improvement. The roots of the current performance or quality-improvement systems can be found in the works of Deming and Major (as discussed in Sashkin & Kiser, 1993). Major national and international quality-management systems share many common elements based on these systems. Some examples follow.

The International Organization for Standardization (ISO; 2003) has published quality-management system standards. The *ISO 9000* system identifies eight principles: customer focus, leadership, involvement of people, process approach, systems approach to management, continual improvement, factual approach to decision making, and supplier relationship.

The *Six Sigma* (Pyzdek, 2003) methodology for improvement is data driven and is designed to help eliminate defects and mistakes in manufacturing and service settings. The six sigma objective is to reduce mistakes and defects to fewer than 3.4 per million opportunities. A defect is defined as any event or outcome that does not meet customer specifications. The sigma system includes the following processes: define, measure, analyze, design (improve), and verify.

The U.S. National Institute of Standards and Technology has established the Baldrige National Quality Program (2005) to promote organizational performance excellence. The core values and concepts of the Baldrige program are found in seven categories: leadership; strategic planning; customer and market focus; measurement, analysis, and knowledge; human resource focus; process management; and business results.

The Balanced Scorecard approach (Kaplan, 1996) to strategic management and quality-improvement requires the development of metrics, data collection, and data analysis to explore the organization from different perspectives: learning and growth, business process, customer, and financial.

These contemporary quality-management and -performance and quality-improvement systems emphasize a focus on the customer. They also stress using a system of metrics that enables the organization to make decisions based on (a) an analysis of data and information concerning outcomes for the customer, and (b) organizational processes that facilitate those outcomes.

An integrated, person-focused QOL outcome system can provide these organizational metrics. It connects the person-centered planning process with a design of organizational processes and supports that facilitate the outcomes. It also provides the integrated metrics that (a) are anchored in the reality of the person-centered planning process, and (b) measure the success of those processes, the status of basic assurances within the organization, and the aggregate quality of life for people served at the support, organizational, or systems level.

An integrated personal outcome measurement system meets the data and information requirements of any quality-management and performance-improvement system. This integrated system provides the range of metrics for quality-management and -performance and quality improvement from both the personal and the systems perspective.

Accreditation

Numerous accreditation programs exist in the fields of health care, education, and service industries. The Joint Commission on Accreditation of Health Care Facilities and the Council on Accreditation provide accreditation programs in the fields of health and human services. CQL, however, is the only organization to design an accreditation program around a set of integrated personal outcome measures. Although many accrediting organizations require the collection and analysis of data, they do not use QOL personal outcome measures as the standard for accreditation. CQL alone accredits organizations based on their success in facilitating the *Personal Outcome Measures* scale.

Summary

The integrated quality system (Figure 5.1) is based on a common set of values and metrics. The framework integrates the functions of quality assurance, quality improvement, and support for quality of life. In addition, the framework leads to coordinated applications in the areas of values alignment, certification of basic assurances, person-directed planning, and the measurement of quality of life for people at the service, organizational, or systems level of application. In addition, the framework of common values and measurement contributes to organizational performance improvement initiatives through internal self-assessment or independent third-party accreditation review.

The integrated quality system works because the same values and measures are used across the system. The person-centered planning, the measurement of the success of that planning, and the assessment of quality of life for people receiving services and supports all rest on the same values and personal outcome measures.

When organizations identify individually defined personal outcomes and aggregate the yes or no responses as to the presence of these outcomes, they can discover a variety of integrated applications. Thus the same quality values and metrics that work at the individual level for each person relate as well to the organizational and systems levels of certification in basic assurances, organizational performance improvement, and accreditation.

The design and development of this integrated quality system reinforces our belief that we can best promote quality by using more meaningful, but less numerous and complex, measures. Based on over two decades of reflection on measurement and quality, we affirm two principles. First, the Pareto Principle, popularized by total quality management gurus in the 1990s, urged us to remember that a relatively small number of variables account for most of the results in any system. This is often translated as 20% of the people do 80% of the work, or 70% of the profit comes from 15% of the production units. Second, more numbers and more measures don't lead to more insight, truth, or enlightenment. Too many numbers and measures often act like weeds and choke off and obscure the flowers we search for in the field.

Quality measures and indicators do not cause either quality of life or quality in services and supports. They enable us to measure and evaluate. We also need measures and indicators that provide information about individuals, are connected to organizational strategy and performance, and provide leadership with information about how to make organizational change. In addition, we need to recognize that organizations exist and function within large systems that have a direct impact on organizational policies and practices. It is to the systems-level considerations of personal outcomes and performance indicators that we now turn.

PART 3

The Systems Perspective

The use of personal outcomes at the systems level needs to be understood within the context of recent legislative and legal trends impacting the services and supports provided to people with intellectual and developmental disabilities (ID-DD). For example, the intent of recent federal legislation has been to ensure the rights to education and community living, access to rehabilitation and employment options and opportunities, technological supports and assistive technology, and person-centered planning. Similarly, legal trends have moved the legal process from (a) dictation to self-determination, (b) exclusion to inclusion, (c) segregation to community-based supports, (d) discrimination to nondiscrimination, and (e) "paper rights" to substantial statutory rights (Herr, O'Sullivan, & Hogan, 2002). Each of these trends, along with the emphasis on accountability and systems efficiency, has forced service-delivery systems to develop systems-level performance indicators that reflect personal outcomes.

Basic to this process has been (a) the development of quality of life (QOL) models based on core quality domains, (b) the focus of activities on the larger system, and (c) the use of personal outcomes for policy analysis and system change. The three chapters in part 3 discuss how the larger system is approaching these three tasks and in the process is conceptualizing, measuring, and using performance indicators and personal outcomes as the basis for quality improvement, policy analysis, and systems change.

Chapter 6 discusses the rationale for using performance indicators that reflect personal outcomes at the system and policy level. Key themes include the movement from the institution, the emergence of individualized supports, person-centered planning, and more recently consumer-driven and directed service and individualized funding. The chapter also addresses changes in oversight at the state and federal level including upgraded quality expectations for states administering the Home and Community-Based Services (HCBS) Waiver Program and the recently proposed HCBS Quality Framework. The chapter discusses the four factors impacting the rationale and need for systems-level performance indicators: (a) the emphasis on quality of life,

(b) changes in social policy and the emergence of performance indicators, (c) significant changes in the service delivery system, and (d) the increasing need for accountability and quality improvement.

Chapter 7 asks the reader to consider the process involved in the development and measurement of macro-level performance indicators. Four important considerations are described: (a) identifying important system trends, (b) delineating positive accomplishments, (c) communicating outcomes to key constituencies, and (d) providing crucial information for managing complex systems. The chapter goes on to lay out a systematic process for developing performance indictors including the involvement of stakeholders, selection of indicators, identification of existing measures and data sources, psychometric review and analysis, design of data collection tools, and risk adjustment of the data to ensure comparability across jurisdictions. The material presented in the chapter builds on—and is complementary to—that presented in previous chapters regarding (a) criteria for reviewing and selecting performance indicators, (b) psychometric properties of personal outcome measures or performance indicators, and (c) risk adjustment and benchmark procedures.

Chapter 8 asks a very basic question: What do you do with the information? It includes a discussion of the development of quality-management committees and the use of a variety of strategies to increase the transparency of quality data including posting quality information on the Web. Guidelines focus on: (a) basing systems for measuring results on a broad commitment to customer service and civic mission, (b) committing oneself to improve performance rather than a set of rules that employees might fear will be used to evaluate them and assign punishment, and (c) establishing reasonable expectations about what results should be measured through consultation with outside overseers.

Throughout these three chapters, the reader will find core concepts and procedures that were part of our discussion of quality outcomes from the individual and organizational perspectives. Chief among these are (a) the need for a conceptual QOL system for an integrated approach to the development and evaluation of performance indicators that reflect personal outcomes, (b) the grounding of that approach in sound measurement principles and procedures, and (c) the need to align values, person-centered planning, personal outcome measurement, person-focused basic assurances, and organizational or system performance improvement.

Terminology will be slightly different in part 3. *Performance indicators,* rather than *personal outcomes,* will be the predominant term used. Performance indicators are a comprehensive set of indicators at the organizational or systems level that typically include (a) aggregate personal outcomes, and (b) other indicators, such as staff turnover, annual medical and dental examinations, and mortality or injury rates. Just as with personal outcomes, performance indicators can be aggregated at the provider and/or systems level *and* complemented by other systems-level indicators. In addition, performance indicators can be analyzed within the context of quality improvement work. It is important to point out that at the systems level, one is not comparing individual definitions of personal outcomes or one program with another; rather, one is measuring the accomplishments of a set of personal outcomes from the system's perspective.

CHAPTER 6

Rationale for Systems-Level Performance Indicators That Reflect Personal Outcomes

Introduction and Overview

Public authorities at the state and substate levels are responsible for the management of systems of services and supports for people with intellectual and developmental disabilities (ID-DD). A critical aspect of this responsibility is the assurance that such services provide value for money spent, meet the needs of the individuals and families who receive them, and are in keeping with statutory and policy expectations. The state, in carrying out its role as system overseer, is functioning in a variety of roles, including purchaser of services, designated regulator of services, and a guardian for the well-being of people served.

Beginning in the 1990s, public managers in the field of ID-DD have been pressed to develop measurement systems that provide a comprehensive and timely picture of services and supports statewide as well as the collection of outcomes for the individuals served by these systems. This pressure has been due in large part to four factors that underlie the need for performance indicators. These four, as discussed in this chapter, are (a) the emphasis on quality of life and personal outcomes, (b) a change in social policy that has included opportunity development for people with ID-DD as reflected in performance indicators, (c) changes in the service delivery system, and (d) an increased emphasis on accountability.

Figure 6.1 depicts these four factors and suggests the key role they play in the need for performance indicators. When reading this chapter, keep in mind these key aspects:

- The quality of life (QOL) concept has influenced the service delivery system through its emphasis on quality services, personal outcomes, and quality improvement.

- The emphasis on performance indicators reflects, in part, both a change in social policy and the complexion of state systems that have become increasingly complex, dispersed, and diverse. As these systems have become more complex, the

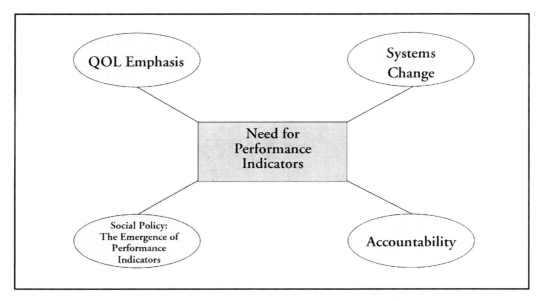

Figure 6.1. Factors influencing the need for systems-level performance indicators.

corresponding need has emerged to (a) monitor these systems regarding performance, trends, and impending problems, and (b) develop evidence-based models to evaluate personal outcomes and implement quality improvement.

• The increased emphasis on accountability at the federal and state levels, which involves policy makers and legislators asking managers to show evidence (a) of the effectiveness of public-funded services, and (b) how performance indicators are used for remediation and quality improvement.

QOL Emphasis

The QOL concept was discussed in chapter 1, with its emphasis on personal outcomes discussed in chapters 2–5. There is no reason to repeat that discussion except to reiterate the evolutionary nature of the concept and how that evolution has impacted the emergence and use of performance indicators. Three aspects of its evolutionary nature are important to readers of this chapter. The first relates to the conceptualization of quality of life. As discussed in part 1, there is a widely accepted consensus that quality of life (a) is multidimensional (see Tables 2.3–2.6), (b) is influenced by personal and environmental factors and their interactions, (c) has the same components for all people, (d) has both subjective and objective components, (e) is measurable, and (f) is enhanced by self-determination, resources, purpose in life, and a sense of belonging.

The second aspect relates to the measurement of quality of life that (a) involves the degree to which people have life experiences that they value; (b) reflects the domains that contribute to a full and interconnected life; (c) considers the context of physical, social, and cultural environments that are important to people; and (d) includes measures of experiences that are both common to all humans and those unique to individuals.

The third aspect relates to the evolution of the concept itself. This evolution is parallel in many aspects to the evolution of performance indicators. For example, historically the QOL concept was used primarily as a sensitizing notion that during the 1980s and 1990s gave us a reference and guidance as to what is valued and desired from the individual's perspective. During the past decade, its roles have expanded to include (a) a conceptual framework for assessing personal outcomes, (b) a social construct that guides quality-improvement efforts, and (c) a criterion for assessing the effectiveness of those efforts.

Social Policy: The Evolution of Performance Indicators

The modern conduct of performance monitoring began in the decades following World War II and grew out of a nationwide institutional reform movement that was manifest in numerous class-action law suits that challenged deplorable conditions in public institutions. As discussed by Bradley and Kimmich (2003):

> These cases, premised on a right to treatment or a right to habilitation, included remedies that prescribed standards for public facilities that had previously been only weakly regulated by the states. Prominent cases included *Wyatt v. Stickney, New York State Association for Retarded Children and Parisi v. Rockefeller* (Willowbrook), *Welsh v. Likens,* and *Davis v. Watkins.* (p. 4)

This rudimentary approach to quality measurement entailed an examination of "inputs" or the basic infrastructure of the facility including physical plant issues, shift schedules, nutrition, and staffing ratios for specific professionals. The approach, while creating some improvement in institutional conditions, was overtaken in the 1970s by a pronounced focus on the "process" or method of service provision. This change coincided with the beginnings of a network of community services and supports and the identification of behavioral, pharmacological, and instructional therapies and interventions. The promise of these approaches prompted federal and state regulators to develop highly prescriptive standards, to ensure that best practices were widely disseminated. These regulations and policies covered things such as the format for individual habilitation plans, the composition of the planning team, and the methods for measuring goal attainment. Concentration on treatment strategies and planning concerns were especially evident in the design of the original regulations governing the conduct of intermediate care facilities for people with mental retardation (ICF-MR) (Bradley & Kimmich, 2003).

These emerging practices became embedded over time in the rapidly expanding community system. This provoked public administrators as well as advocates to expand their performance expectations beyond inputs and process to an examination of outcomes. Using functional scales, such as the Scales of Independent Behavior (Bruininks, Hill, Weatherman, & Woodcock, 1986) and the Vineland Adaptive Behavior Scales (Sparrow, Balla, & Cicchetti, 1984), initial outcome measures were tied to the achievement of specific learning or behavioral benchmarks, such as cooking, taking public transit, and reduction in maladaptive behavior.

As community systems continued to mature and as notions of community inclusion and individual empowerment became broadly embraced, public managers were pressed to include the expectations of individuals and families in the design of outcome and performance monitoring. (For a current discussion of these expectations, see Swenson [2005].) The most dramatic example of this shift was the substantially revamped standards published by the Accreditation Council on Services for People With Disabilities (ACD; 1993). Eschewing the complex set of process standards that had previously been the hallmark of ACD, the accrediting body adopted a set of nine valued outcomes: choice, social inclusion, relationships, rights, dignity and respect, health, environment, security, and satisfaction.

This increasing emphasis on outcomes in performance assessment was more than merely a change in measurement approaches. It reflected both the evolution of process to outcomes and the use of logic models that emphasize the impact of external factors on human service programs. More specifically, the emphasis on outcomes represented a change from professionally dictated, programmatic models of oversight to a more democratic approach to quality that has reshaped practice by placing the experience of the individual in the center of the analysis.

Systems Change

Expansion and Dispersal of Services and Supports

Community services and supports have expanded rapidly over the past three decades. According to the most recent report from the Institute on Community Integration in Minnesota (Prouty, Smith, & Lakin, 2005), the number of residential settings for people with ID-DD is growing rapidly. On June 30, 2003, there were an estimated 145,581 residential settings.

> Since 1977, the number of such settings has grown more than thirteen-fold. In comparison, on June 30, 1977 there were 11,008 state licensed or state operated residential service settings; on June 30, 1987 there were 33,477; on June 30, 1992 there were 49,479; on June 30, 1995 there were 84,532; and on June 30, 1998 there were 104,765. (p. iv)

Most of these residences were small and managed primarily by private for-profit and nonprofit organizations. On June 30, 2004, an estimated 144,460 (99.2%) residences had 15 or fewer residents and 140,584 (95.3%) had 6 or fewer residents. Further, the number of people served in dispersed residential settings has also skyrocketed. The total population increases can be solely attributed to the expansion of facilities with 15 or fewer residents. In those settings the populations increased from 247,780 in 1977 to 420,200 in 2004 (Prouty et al., 2005). It is also important to note that there has been a significant increase in the number of people with ID-DD receiving supports at home.

These numbers provide dramatic evidence that public overseers are severely taxed in their ability to conduct frequent onsite monitoring at the myriad sites where people are receiving residential supports. In addition, there has also been a significant growth in the HCBS Waiver Program and the expansion of managed care.

Growth of the Home and Community-Based Waiver

During the 1990s, there was a massive expansion in the Medicaid HCBS Waiver Program for people with developmental disabilities. According to Prouty et al. (2005), as of June 30, 2003,

> there were 402,438 persons with intellectual and other developmental disabilities receiving HCBS, an increase of 6.3% over 378,566 recipients on June 30, 2002. In the thirteen years between June 30, 1990 and 2003, the number of HCBS recipients grew by 362,600 persons (910.2%) from 39,838 HCBS recipients. (p. vii)

The number of individuals in such programs increased from roughly 45,000 in 1990 to 291,000 in 2000 (Smith, O'Keefe, Carpenter, Dota, & Kennedy, 2000). States anticipated that they would be expected to collect and report more robust information concerning the quality and effectiveness of home and community services. These expectations were subsequently proven correct when the Health Care Financing Administration released its waiver quality protocol (U.S. Department of Health & Human Services, 2000).

Expansion of Managed Care

In the early 1990s, it seemed that many states would radically restructure not only their health and behavioral health care, but also other long-term services systems along managed-care lines. Although this was cause for concern, it prompted officials in many states to take a fresh look at how they were managing their systems, especially with regard to the type of data-based system management employed in managed care. Public managers in ID-DD saw that emerging data-based indicators were viable, and they started to think proactively about the importance of pursuing a set of indicators with particular relevance to their constituency (Human Services Research Institute &

National Association of State Directors of Developmental Disabilities Services, 2003).

Growth of Performance Indicators in Other Fields

It is important to note that the movement to performance indicators in the ID-DD field was preceded by a similar movement in the field of behavioral health. Some of this work was associated with the emergence of managed health care (e.g., Health Plan Employer Data Information Set; National Committee on Quality Assurance, 2006). In the 1990s several efforts were underway in behavioral health to develop and implement performance indicators, including in the public sector (e.g., Mental Health Statistics Improvement Program; National Institute of Mental Health, 1989) and American Academy of Mental Health Administrators performance indicators (Sante Fe Summit, 1997). This work strongly suggested the potential for developing performance indicators for developmental disabilities services.

Importance of Data-Driven Policies

As state systems of services and supports have become increasingly complex, dispersed, and diverse, the need for performance indicators has become apparent. To monitor these systems in the absence of any significant onsite capability, public managers require valid, reliable, and illustrative data regarding performance, trends, and impending problems. Further, not simply satisfied with preventing crises or identifying vulnerabilities, public managers have also become interested in enhancing the quality of state and substate systems through technical assistance, policy change, and propagation of best practice. Quality improvement initiatives are highly dependent on data that identify trends and effective practice (U.S. Department of Health & Human Services, 2003).

Increasing Consensus About What Constitutes Quality

This systems change has been accompanied by an acrimonious debate regarding the downsizing of public institutions and the expansion of community services. Although some of this debate continues in particular states (e.g., IL & MA), the intensity of the argument has subsided. This is in large measure due to the continual decline in institutional populations. Between fiscal years 1980 and 2003, the average daily population of large state facilities decreased by 87,799 (67%) to 43,289 individuals. During that same period, 41 states reduced their institutional census by 50% or more (Prouty et al., 2005).

As the debate about institutions has receded, the basic assumptions about expected outcomes for people and systems are increasingly shared across multiple stakeholders. The outcomes initially advanced by ACD in 1993 (see updated domains and indicators in Table 2.5) are now arguably the basic governing tenets of the field. As a consequence, the ability to gain support for a core set of indicators that represent the views of consumers, providers, families, advocates, and administrators is substantially enhanced.

Pressure for Accountability

Three examples of the increased emphasis on accountability are discussed below.

Government Performance and Reporting Act of 1993

Over the past several years, there has been increasing emphasis on accountability at the federal and state levels as policy makers and legislators are asking managers to show evidence of the effectiveness of publicly funded services. This emphasis on proven efficacy in the federal government was strongly reinforced with the passage of the Government Performance and Results Act of 1993 (GPRA). GPRA requires executive branch managers to set goals more systematically, measure performance against goals, and make public reports on their progress toward goals. The law specifically requires that, as part of Program Performance Reports, each agency must establish performance indicators to be used in measuring or assessing the relevant outputs, service levels, and outcomes of each program activity.

Federal Program Assessment Rating Tool

More recently the U.S. Office of Management and Budget (2002) has initiated the Program Assessment Rating Tool (PART) to assess the effectiveness of specific federal programs and to help inform management actions, budget requests, and legislative proposals directed at achieving results. The PART examines factors that contribute to the effectiveness of a program; it requires that conclusions be explained and substantiated with evidence. The PART assesses if and how program evaluation is used to inform program planning and to corroborate program results. Although there are no explicit connections between GPRA and PART, they are obviously connected insofar as the intent of each is to amplify accountability.

Relating Costs to Outcomes

Another aspect of increased accountability involves relating costs and outcomes of community services for people with ID-DD. As discussed in the foreword to Stancliffe and Lakin (2005), Eidelman stresses that much of our efforts to date have focused on obtaining funds to support people in the community. He then points out that,

> we are in the process of transitioning to a system that supports people who may or may not purchase those supports from organizations historically involved in providing paid supports for people with ID/DD: a transition to a market economy . . . [where] consumers have data about costs, quality, and outcomes. (p. xxvii)

A detailed discussion of attempts to relate costs to outcomes can be found in Stancliffe and Lakin (2005) and in Schalock (2001).

These three accountability initiatives have been mirrored at the state level. Examples include the creation of performance indicators in Vermont to monitor the state's consumer-driven funding mechanism, the launch of the Quality Outcomes Project in New Hampshire, and the initiation of the National Core Indicators (NCI) by state ID-DD managers in 1997 (Human Services Research Institute & National Association of State Directors of Developmental Disabilities Services, 2003). All these initiatives have enhanced the ability of states to ensure that services and supports are accountable to people with developmental disabilities, their families, and the taxpayer. These and analogous state initiatives will be discussed further in chapter 8.

Changes in Federal Expectations

Community services and supports for people with ID-DD are funded substantially through federal HCBS waivers. As a result, the administrators of the program at the U.S. Centers for Medicare and Medicaid Services (CMS) have gradually developed more specific expectations regarding what constitutes quality in HCBS. These expectations have been influenced in part by problems in waiver reviews in the 1990s and the U.S. General Accounting Office (GAO) critique of CMS monitoring.

Problems in Waiver Reviews in the 1990s

In the late 1990s and early 2000s, a number of states, including California, Illinois, Ohio, and Tennessee, were found to have serious problems in the implementation of their HCBS waivers, problems that potentially jeopardized the health and safety of waiver recipients. A recent review of 13 state waiver reports found the following major clusters of citations (Rowe & Taub, 2002):

- *Provider capabilities,* including staff training or workforce development and development of coordinated and effective systems to monitor providers

- *Service planning and implementation,* particularly regarding increased choice among providers and services

- *Participant safeguards,* predominantly regarding health and medication

- *Systems monitoring and performance,* particularly the development of cohesive quality management and quality assurance systems with more specific data collection and dissemination protocols

In response, CMS has revamped its HCBS Waiver Program review protocol (U.S. Department of Health & Human Services, 2002). The protocol encourages states to collect systematic performance and outcome data along several dimensions, including satisfaction with services. CMS also commissioned the development of a Participant Experience Survey (U.S. Department of Health & Human Services, 2003) that collects data on outcomes for individual waiver participants.

GAO Critique of CMS Monitoring

In 2003, the U.S. GAO evaluated the monitoring of state HCBS programs conducted by CMS regional employees. This evaluation found that:

- CMS provides no detailed guidance to states on the necessary components of a quality assurance system for HCBS.

- States provide limited information about quality approaches in annual reports to CMS.

- Quality issues have been identified in HCBS waiver reviews.

- CMS reviews are not conducted in a timely fashion.

These 2003 findings lent a sense of immediacy to the emerging and expanding quality initiatives at CMS and resulted in the development of the Quality Framework and interim procedural guidance and new waiver application process.

Development of the Quality Framework

In August 2002 CMS circulated a memo that introduced a comprehensive model for organizing the components of a quality assurance system. The Quality Framework, presented in Figure 6.2, was initially designed to organize the results of a 50-state

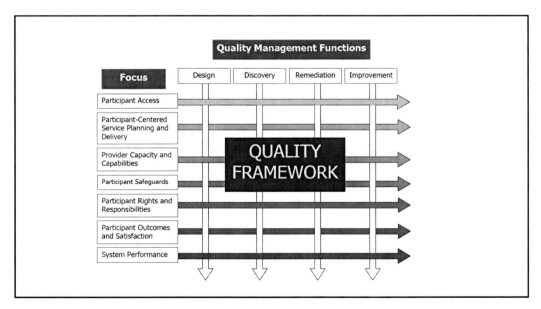

Figure 6.2. U.S. Centers for Medicare and Medicaid Services, quality framework for home and community-based services.

Note. From *Quality Letters* (1–9). U.S. Department of Health and Human Services, Centers for Medicare and Medicaid Services. 2005. Retrieved October 5, 2005, from https://cms.hhs.gov/medicaid/waiversqcomm.asp.

inventory of HCBS quality assurance practices. The framework is organized both in terms of quality assurance components and the functions that should be aligned with each component, including design, discovery (data collection), remediation (use of data to respond to immediate problems), and improvement (use of data to improve services and supports at the systems level). This framework is being used by many state HCBS Waiver Programs to evaluate their quality assurance systems to ensure that they include all requisite components and functions.

Interim Procedural Guidance and New Waiver Application

The most recent initiatives launched by CMS that will also influence the ways states organize and report quality assurance information are (a) the circulation of Interim Procedural Guidance, which lays out an "evidence-based" template for reporting quality assurance data, and (b) the development of a new application for the HCBS waiver, which incorporates many of the aspects of the Quality Framework and the Interim Procedural Guidance, and specifies how states will keep CMS and its regional offices informed of quality findings, trends, and quality improvement actions.

This flurry of activity at the CMS has made it clear that states will be expected to collect and report more robust information concerning the quality and effectiveness of home and community services. This expectation underscores the rationale for systems-level performance indicators that reflect personal outcomes.

Summary

As discussed in this chapter, the emergence of systems-level performance indicators in public ID-DD systems is part of an evolutionary process that parallels the growth of community supports and services, the increasing participation of the federal government in funding such services, a consensus regarding the aspects of performance worthy of measurement, and an increased sophistication among public managers regarding the prerequisites of quality management and improvement efforts. The emergence of performance indicators has not occurred in a vacuum. Indeed, as shown in Figure 6.1 and discussed in this chapter, the rationale and use of systems-level performance indicators that reflect personal outcomes has been influenced significantly by four factors: (a) the emphasis on quality of life, (b) a social policy that requires performance indicators, (c) changes in the service delivery system, and (d) the need for accountability in the process and outcomes of services and supports.

In addition to those measurement principles and procedures discussed in chapter 3, the following chapter will discuss the development and measurement of quality indicators at the macro level. Throughout that discussion keep two things in mind: (a) Multiple stakeholders are interested in performance indicators that reflect personal outcomes; and (b) the evaluation requirements, information, and reports are numerous. The plethory of data and the possibility that some systems are data rich and information poor point to the need for three evaluation and reporting standards to ensure accuracy and credibility of information (Schwartz & Mayne, 2005):

- *Product quality:* well-defined scope, systematic (e.g., organized, sequential, logical), accurate data, sound analysis, impartial or objective findings and conclusions
- *Process quality:* involves key stakeholders, being transparent, and being an ongoing part of services and supports provision
- *Information usefulness:* timeliness (i.e., the information is produced at a time when it can make a difference in improving the organization's performance), relevant in scope (i.e., the information produced is relevant to the issues of the day), and clarity (i.e., the information is understandable by the intended audience(s)

Systems performance indicators that reflect personal outcomes are the basis for program accountability. Used properly, they not only validate services and supports, but they also provide key information in the quality improvement process. That concept will be discussed further in part 4. In the next chapter we look at considerations in developing indicators at the macro level.

CHAPTER 7

Considerations in Developing Performance Indicators at the Macro Level

Introduction and Overview

The previous chapter described the emergence of performance measurement as a key facet of federal and state oversight of services and supports to people with intellectual and developmental disabilities (ID-DD). In this chapter we will describe the policy, methodological, and practical considerations that frame any performance measurement construct at the system (i.e., federal, state, substate, and provider) levels.

To respond to our heterogeneous readership, composed of researchers, evaluators, program managers, policy makers, and systems managers, we will continue to use clearly defined terms and concepts, principles, and guidelines that go across the micro, meso, and macro systems and provide specific examples taken from our collective efforts. In this chapter we will refer to the National Core Indicators that arose initially in response to the changing service delivery system's increased complexity and the need for accountability discussed in the previous chapter.

The material presented in this chapter builds on—and is complementary to—that presented in previous chapters. Specifically, the criteria for reviewing and selecting performance indicators in this chapter are essentially the same as presented in Table 2.8, except here they reflect additional systems-level considerations. Similarly the psychometric properties discussed herein are the same as those presented in Table 3.3 but referenced to the larger macro system with its unique characteristics. Finally, the discussion of risk adjustment, norms, and benchmarks expands significantly on the "reporting issues" addressed in chapter 3. Our discussion in chapter 3 regarding the use of proxies and their impact also applies to this chapter, because proxies are used frequently in systems-level data collection centering on performance indicators that reflect personal outcomes.

The chapter begins with an overview of the National Core Indicators and describes their rationale, development, and use. (This description provides the basis for much of the material presented in the remaining sections of the chapter.) Thereafter, we discuss the purpose of systems-level performance indicators. Our discussion then proceeds to selecting indicators, identifying and reviewing existing measures and data sources, conducting psychometric tests of the measures, designing data collection tools, selecting the final measures, and developing norms and benchmarks. The chapter concludes with a discussion of the outcome from these efforts and the usefulness of the resulting information.

National Core Indicators

Background
In January 1977 the National Association of State Directors of Developmental Disabilities Services (NASDDDS) and the Human Services Research Institute (HSRI) launched the National Core Indicators (NCI). The number of participating states has climbed steadily, reaching 22 in the spring of 2004 (plus the Regional Center of Orange County, CA). The decision to initiate NCI grew out of the recognition by the members of NASDDDS that the increasing complexity of ID-DD services required vastly improved capabilities to evaluate overall system performance. State officials also recognized that quality improvement hinges on the capacity to conduct systematic and rigorous measurements of performance and outcomes. Absent such measures, it is virtually impossible to design and implement meaningful improvement strategies. Moreover, member agencies also recognized the importance of being able to furnish performance information to state funders and other system stakeholders. NCI continues to be a voluntary collaboration among participating NASDDDS member agencies and substate entities. Participating states pool their resources and knowledge to create performance monitoring systems, identify common performance indicators, work out sound data collection strategies, and share results.

Consumer Survey
The NCI consumer survey (HSRI, 2004) was initially developed by the project's technical advisory subcommittee with the purpose of collecting information directly from individuals with ID-DD and their families or advocates regarding outcomes such as choice, relationships, personal safety, transportation, and community participation. The survey is designed to measure more than half of the 60 core indicators (see Tables 2.6 & 7.2). Project staff have tested and refined the instrument each year based on feedback from interviewers. Currently NCI has a national database comprising almost 10,000 consumer responses. Data in Table 7.1 show, for example, the percentage of respondents saying yes to each core indicator listed.

States use a variety of types of surveyors, including consumers and families, university students, and state personnel. Some independent interviewers are paid; others are volunteers (unpaid). These methods have been acceptable; no major

Table 7.1

Percentage of Respondents Answering "Yes" to National Core Indicators

Core Indicator	% Yes
People choose where to live.	53.0
People choose whom to live with.	45.0
People choose where they work.	62.1
People have friends (not staff or family).	68.0
People have close friends.	85.5
People like where they live.	89.2
People like where they work.	91.1
People get help to do new things.	75.6
People have transportation.	81.7
People get the services they need.	80.5
People go shopping.	93.6
People go out on errands.	96.3
People go out for entertainment.	86.0
People go out to eat.	92.5
People go to religious services.	57.4
People go out to clubs or community meetings.	29.3
People exercise in nonintegrated settings.	34.2
People read own mail.	80.7
People can be alone with guests.	75.2
People can use the phone any time.	87.4
People can be alone (can have privacy).	92.8

Note. N = 9,192. Data from *National Core Indicators: 5 Years of Performance Measurement,* by Human Services Research Institute & National Association of State Directors of Developmental Disabilities Services, 2003, Cambridge, MA, & Alexandria, VA. Used with permission.

differences in survey results have been noted in terms of types of interviewers. One stipulation has been made—that if case managers conduct interviews, they do not interview consumers on their own caseload.

Other Protocols
In addition to the consumer survey, there are other protocols for soliciting data on a

range of systems and provider issues (e.g., serious injuries, staff stability) as well as on family perceptions of outcomes for the family unit and for the family member with a disability (HSRI, 2004; HSRI & NASDDDS, 2003).

Purposes of System-Level Performance Indicators

Data-based performance information can be used for a number of purposes, including (a) identifying trends, (b) illuminating positive accomplishments, (c) communicating outcomes to key constituencies, and (d) providing crucial information for managing complex systems.

Identifying Trends

Several performance indicators, in addition to personal outcomes as discussed in parts 1 and 2, when tracked systematically can alert public managers about incipient and or looming changes in the conduct of the system, thus requiring either immediate remediation or long-term interventions. For example, creating trend data to analyze mortality can yield information on unexpected deaths and cause of death, which, in turn, can stimulate policy and training initiatives. If deaths from sepsis and aspiration pneumonia are increasing, this information may suggest that direct-support professionals are insufficiently trained to identify symptoms or that access to health care has been compromised.

Illuminating Positive Accomplishments

Performance indicators can also be used to determine trends that suggest positive accomplishments. Using information to highlight outcomes, such as improvements in health status, reduction in abuse and neglect substantiations, or increases in choice and self-determination, can help public managers identify and replicate successful programs. The circulation of positive results can also elevate the morale of system managers and providers and show legislators the benefits of public tax investments.

Communicating Outcomes to Key Constituencies

Public ID-DD systems are no longer solely the purview of professionals and public managers. Over the years, and as a result of the family support movement, the self-advocacy movement, and the more recent embrace of self-determination, "ownership" of services and supports to people with ID-DD is now shared broadly across multiple constituencies. To honor the "shareholders" in the system, transparency is critical, and it can be achieved by disseminating performance data. The communication of outcomes can also facilitate joint problem solving and strategic planning across key systemic actors.

Providing Crucial Information for Managing Complex Systems

As noted in the previous chapter, across the country the systems of public support for people with ID-DD have expanded into highly complex networks composed of widely varying levels and types of providers, settings, and structures. The ability of budget-constrained state managers to maintain even a periodic physical oversight of such far-flung services declines daily. As a consequence, such administrators need more sophisticated and data-driven methods to track system performance. Quality indicators and personal outcomes described previously (see Tables 2.4–2.7 & 7.1) provide the basis for such data-driven methods.

Selecting Performance Indicators

Let's look at two steps in the process of selecting performance indicators.

Establish an Advisory Committee

Any system of indicators that is applied to measure the performance of public disabilities systems needs to have face validity with key stakeholders. The first step in the development of performance indicators should be to form a committee that is representative of the various constituency groups, including advocates, people with ID-DD and their families, and service providers. The primary purpose of this committee is to assure that the indicators are meaningful, that the performance aspirations are reasonable, and that the monitoring systems are economically and administratively feasible.

Managers may want to consider appointing two committees, one to advise on the programmatic content of the indicators, the second to focus on technical issues. People in the second group should have experience with the technical issues involved in the development of performance-monitoring systems. It is their job to match the indicators with existing data sources and to assure that the resulting performance-monitoring system is technically sound.

Review Preliminary Performance Indicators

The next step is to develop, with the assistance of the stakeholder panel, a list of candidate performance indicators. Based on experience with the NCI effort, the process is greatly aided by circulation of potential performance indicators gleaned from the literature and from other public entities. In addition to the potential indicators listed in Table 2.4, Table 7.2 summarizes performance indicators reflecting the quality of life (QOL)-related domains of system performance; health, welfare, and rights; staff stability and competence; family issues; and case management. (Detailed descriptions of these domains and their respective concerns, which in turn translate into indicators, are found in HSRI & NASDDDS, 2003.)

Having access to these multidimensional performance indicators improves the efficiency of the group process and facilitates an understanding of the characteristics of indicators across individuals, organizations, and the service delivery system. The

	TABLE 7.2	
	Potential Performance Indicators That Reflect Personal Outcomes	
Domain	**Subdomain**	**Concern**
System performance	Service coordination	Service coordinators are accessible, responsive, and support the person's participation in service planning.
	Family and individual participation	Families and individuals are involved in provider-level decision making.
	The service system supports community integration and personal independence.	Use of selected service(s)
	Financial level of efforts	There are sufficient dollars to meet the needs of individuals.
	Cultural competency	Racial and ethnic minorities have access to services and supports.
	Access	Publicly funded services are readily available to individuals who need and qualify for them.
Health, welfare, and rights	Safety	People are safe from abuse, neglect, and injury.
	Health	People secure needed health services.
	Medications	Medications are managed effectively and appropriately.
	Wellness	People are supported to maintain healthy habits
	Restraints	The system makes limited use of restraints or other restrictive practices.
	Respect or rights	People receive the same respect and protections as others in the community.

(table continues)

TABLE 7.2 *(continued)*		
Domain	**Subdomain**	**Concern**
Staff stability and competence	Staff stability	Direct-contact staff turnover ratios and recruitment and training absentee rates are low enough to maintain continuity of supports and efficient use of resources.
	Staff competence	Direct-contact staff members are competent to provide services and supports.
Family issues	Information and planning	Families and family members with disabilities have the information and support necessary to plan for their services and supports.
	Choice and control	Families and family members with disabilities determine the services and supports they receive and the individuals or agencies that provide them.
	Access and support delivery	Families and family members with disabilities get the services and supports they need.
	Community connections	Families and family members use integrated community services and participate in everyday community activities.
	Family involvement	Families maintain connections with family members not living at home.
	Satisfaction	Families and family members with disabilities receive adequate and satisfactory supports.
	Family outcomes	Individual and family supports make a positive difference in the lives of families.

(table continues)

TABLE 7.2 *(continued)*		
Domain	Subdomain	Concern
Case management	Skills	Is staff knowledgeable, adequately trained, and confident in abilities?
	Values	Does staff support the values held by the state Developmental Disabilities Authority?

list can be organized by domains such as health and safety, choice and self-determination, community inclusion, and employment.

Another way of proceeding, which requires careful facilitation, is to work with the group to develop a *de novo* set of performance indicators. This requires helping the group through a series of questions and reflections on program goals (e.g., people make choices, people get jobs, people are safe) and then identifying how the system would know that the goal had been achieved. There are several criteria for indicators developed by this process.

1. Indicators should reflect the *mission* of the organization.

2. Indicators should be *clinically or programmatically useful*. They should address outcomes or processes that are of central concern to the quality of life and the health and safety of people with ID-DD who receive services and supports.

3. The set of indicators should be *comprehensive in scope*. Indicators should address a comprehensive array of outcomes; they should also provide evidence and data that will be useful at the state level and satisfy the state legislature, the federal Centers for Medicare and Medicaid Services, and other oversight and regulatory bodies.

4. The set of indicators should be *minimally redundant* with respect to content.

5. The indicators should reflect phenomena that are *neither too rare nor too common*. If the phenomenon is too rare, it won't occur frequently enough or in sufficient numbers to identify trends and reasonable benchmarks. If it is too common, the phenomenon may not show sufficient change or fluctuation.

6. The indicators should address outcomes or processes over which the public ID-DD system administrators have some *control*. If the indicators measure events that are outside the purview of the agency, any resulting poor outcomes can only serve to frustrate and demoralize the organization.

The stakeholder group should be instructed to weigh the above criteria as members assemble a list of potential indicators that is somewhat larger than what is expected to be included in the final set. Some indicators will likely prove too difficult or costly to operationalize and will ultimately be dropped from the set.

Identifying and Reviewing Existing Measures and Data Sources

Once the initial pool of performance indicators has been selected, the technical group needs to identify measures that are aligned with each potential indicator and develop quantifiable statements that capture the outcome anticipated by the indicator (e.g., the proportion of people who have jobs, the proportion of people who feel safe in their communities). The possible measures associated with each indicator should be analyzed by the technical panel through a structured process to ensure that every measure meets acceptable standards of scientific integrity. Use the following list of selection criteria to judge the adequacy of each potential performance measure or personal outcome:

1. The measures should have demonstrated *reliability*. This refers to the stability of measures over repeated measurements (test-retest reliability) and across different raters (interrater reliability).

2. In the case of multi-item scales, the items must be *internally consistent*.

3. The measures must be *valid*. They should (a) demonstrate the ability to detect differences in quality of services across different organizations, (b) be capable of detecting differences among consumer groups or among organizations that are hypothesized to vary with respect to the outcomes of interest (*discriminant validity*), and (c) be highly correlated with other measures hypothesized to be measuring the same construct (*concurrent validity*).

4. The measures should reflect phenomena that have the potential of differentiating among elements such as service settings, geographic areas, and levels of functioning.

5. Taken as a whole, the measures should demonstrate minimal statistical redundancy so that the set is efficient.

6. The level of effort required to compile data and compute scores should not be overly burdensome.

7. The meaning of scores on any single measure or combination of measures should be as unambiguous as possible in terms of its program and policy implications.

To facilitate the review process by the advisory committee, each of the potential measures should also be aligned with existing data sources (e.g., surveys, incident reports, mortality reports), and these data sources should in turn be rated based on the frequency with which they are collected, the level of confidence in the data, and other characteristics that will help the technical group make decisions about viable measures and data sources. This process will also help to identify those measures for which no data are currently collected and will facilitate the creation of new data collection protocols and processes.

Finally, you'll need to identify *specific criteria* that each measure must demonstrate for inclusion in the final set of measures. For example, the committee may decide that measure reliability is so important that any measure without demonstrated reliability should not be included. Members should then be asked to discuss the merits of each measure and data source, in terms of their programmatic importance, psychometric robustness, and feasibility.

You can anticipate that panels will identify three subsets of indicators: (a) those for which already tested and acceptable measures exist (e.g., number of serious incidents reported, frequency of health check-ups), (b) those for which likely measures exist, but the measures require further testing to demonstrate their psychometric strength and/or feasibility (e.g., existing client surveys), and (c) those for which adequate measures do not exist (e.g., indicators of self-determination, social inclusion, or personal development).

Conducting Psychometric Tests of Measures

The next step is to conduct psychometric tests of the new and existing measures for which sufficient psychometric data have not been developed. Appropriate tests of reliability and validity should be conducted depending on the type of measure.

Reliability
Reliability refers to consistency of measurements across time and/or across different raters. All measures (except objective and self-report measures) should be subjected to tests of interrater reliability by having two raters complete each item using the same instrument and the same data sources. Test-retest analyses should be conducted on all self-report items by having each respondent complete each item twice, with testing separated by two weeks. A two-week interval is considered long enough so that respondents typically cannot remember how they answered a particular item, but not so long that most phenomena under study would have changed significantly. Different statistics should be computed, depending on the type of data (see Table 3.3).

Validity
Validity refers to the extent to which an item or set of items measures only the desired construct and is not contaminated with other varying phenomenon. It is considerably more difficult to assess than reliability. Several types of validity, including concurrent or convergent validity, predictive validity, and face validity, should be assessed in regard to performance indicators that reflect personal outcomes.

Concurrent or Convergent Validity

Concurrent or convergent validity refers to how well an item score corresponds to or predicts scores on another psychometrically or clinically sound instrument. For instance, for a particular group, if it is not possible to gather information using a standardized battery of tests, it may be necessary to substitute a less sophisticated and labor-intensive measure. It will be important to measure the concurrent validity of the proposed probe with the score from the standardized instrument.

Predictive Validity

Predictive validity refers to the ability of a scale or item to differentiate among groups of respondents on the basis of known characteristics. For instance, if a measure is intended to measure the intensity of behavioral issues, it should predict between those with known behavioral challenges and those without or those with high versus low behavioral support needs.

Face Validity

Face validity is the determination of whether the measure "on its face" reflects the performance target that is being assessed. For instance, if the targeted outcome is choice, do the proposed measures reflect the ability of individuals to make life choices in a variety of areas including work, and where and with whom they live? In the case of the ID-DD field, it is also important to determine whether measures reflect areas of a program or a system that are of concern to various stakeholders.

Designing Data Collection Tools

Survey Construction and Testing

The primary data source for many of the performance indicators identified by the advisory group will undoubtedly come from the direct reports of individuals and families through the administration of a consumer survey or interview instrument. Unless there is a psychometrically sound survey available, it will be necessary to design an information-gathering instrument.

A number of researchers have pointed to significant administrative and technical problems in obtaining subjective information from people with cognitive disabilities (Andrews & Withey, 1976; Converse & Presser, 1986; Heal & Sigelman, 1996). Numerous methods must be devised and tested to control for the strong tendency of people with cognitive disabilities to respond positively (acquiescent response bias) and to provide socially acceptable responses. Survey instruments must be constructed to minimize or at least detect and account for the known tendency of people with ID-DD to let prior responses color subsequent responses (recency bias). Questions need to be worded well to minimize the need to paraphrase questions, given the known distortions that result (Antaki & Rapley, 1996). Sound protocols should be devised and reviewed for deciding when proxy reports should be used in lieu of self-reports. The development of the consumer survey as part of the NCI (HSRI, 2004) provides an illustrative example of survey construction and testing.

In 1997, once the HSRI identified core indicators that rely on consumer reports, the project team designed a consumer survey or interview instrument that was administered by the original seven field-test states (VT, CT, AZ, PA, NE, VA, & MO). The draft instrument was constructed to capture data for each of the performance indicator measures that required direct client reports. The draft NCI instrument was reviewed by an expert panel of state evaluators and a decision was made to divide the survey into two parts—one part that could be answered only by the individual with ID-DD, and a second section that, if the individual could not answer, could be answered by an advocate, family member, or another closely associated individual. The former included questions that were intersubjective (e.g., "do people treat you with respect?"), and the latter included more instrumental questions (e.g., "does the person need a communication device?"). Further, a focus group was held with individuals with cognitive disabilities, to ensure that the questions were meaningful and understandable.

In November and December 1997, a pilot test of the NCI instrument was conducted, administered to 30 individuals. The purpose of this pilot test was to refine the survey questions and to test interrater reliability. The test confirmed that the instrument had a high level of interrater reliability. The pilot study findings led to further changes in the wording of the questions and to specifications for how interviewers would record responses.

A Field-Test Version of the instrument was prepared and distributed to all the field-test states. Nebraska developmental disabilities managers agreed to conduct a final reliability test in conjunction with their administration of the consumer survey or interview. Training materials and videotapes were developed to ensure consistency of administration.

Once the instrument was finalized, each of the seven states launched its consumer surveys or interviews. A minimum of 400 randomly selected individuals across all service settings were surveyed in each state, beginning in early 1998. Standard consent procedures were followed to obtain agreement from individuals to participate in the survey. Standard protocols were followed to protect the confidentiality of individual responses.

Risk Adjustment

The ability of individuals to achieve outcomes or performance goals (e.g., health, safety, personal growth, and quality of life) is intuitively related to their adaptive skills and capacities. For example, individuals with gross motor limitations are probably more prone to falls and injury than those who do not have such limitations; individuals who are bed-ridden are probably more prone to pressure sores; individuals lacking verbal communication skills are probably less successful in establishing relationships than people with verbal skills. To compare providers, regions, or states using performance indicators, it is important to account for these variations through a process called risk assessment.

Controlling for the effect of these risk factors can be done in two ways. One is to stratify clients into groups having similar risk factors, to permit fair comparisons of like groups. Another is to weight the presence of these risk factors to arrive at an expected rate. This risk-adjusted rate accounts for the different levels of risk in each provider, area, or state and makes possible fair comparisons and interpretations. The stratification approach has been adopted in developing performance indicators both for home health agencies and nursing homes.

The necessity for risk adjustment was apparent in NCI, because one major use for the data was to make state-by-state comparisons. Given the differences in eligible populations across states (i.e., some states serve only people with cognitive disabilities while other states serve a broader developmental disabilities population), it was anticipated that there would be variations in the risk factors. To ensure the comparability of NCI consumer data across states, the first step was to collect information on the functional characteristics of the individuals sampled. Project staff selected the *Inventory for Client and Agency Planning* (ICAP; Bruininks, Hill, Weatherman, & Woodcock, 1986) to obtain this data, given its proven psychometric properties and the broad use of the instrument in the field.

Data from the full ICAP were subsequently analyzed to "risk adjust" the results of the consumer survey and thereby determine the extent to which various consumer outcomes were affected by differences in consumer characteristics. The analysis was conducted in two stages that spanned the initial pilot data collection phase and the first official round of state data collection.

In the first year, NCI staff used a combination of empirical analysis and judgment to identify a subset of consumer characteristics to help assess the use and feasibility of adjusting state outcomes to allow for state differences in consumer mix. The empirical analysis consisted of statistical tests performed on consumers surveyed in the pilot stage. Through these procedures, NCI identified four measures to facilitate outcome adjustment in the first year: age, level of mental retardation, mobility assistance needed, and behavioral problems. Although single questions could be used to measure age, level of mental retardation, level of mobility, and maladaptive behaviors were multidimensional and required multiple questions.

The results in the second year included (a) computing for each core indicator the unadjusted means for each state; (b) running an analysis of variance (ANOVA) test, controlling for the 4 variables identified in the first-year analysis; (c) adding 9 additional demographic variables for a total of 13 and then rerunning the same group of analyses; and (d) ordering the list of 13 variables according to the number of indicators for which the factor was a significant predictor of outcomes (Ashbaugh, Banks, & Taub, 1999). Items shown below in bold were found to be significant in the first-year analysis.

1. **Level of mental retardation**

2. **Currently taking psychoactive or anticonvulsant medications**

3. Additional diagnoses (other than mental retardation)

4. **Age**

5. **Mobility (walks with or without aids, does not walk, limited to bed most of the day, or confined to bed for entire day)**

6. Legal status (legally competent adult, parent or relative guardian, nonrelative guardian, state or county guardian)

7. Frequency of seizures (none, < monthly, monthly, weekly or more than weekly)

8. **Measure of behavior problems (4-item scale)**

9. Gender

10. Required care of nurse or physician (< monthly, monthly, weekly, daily, 24-hour or immediate access)

11. Primary means of expression (none, gestures, speaks, sign language or finger spelling, communication device)

12. Vision (sees well, problems limit reading or travel, little or no useful vision)

13. Race

Selecting Final Measures

Once performance indicators have been developed, measures created and validated, and potential data sources identified, it is important to assess the practical implications of implementing some or all of the components of the performance monitoring scheme. This includes a variety of calculations, including the viability of existing management information systems for analysis, the cost of survey administration, and the likelihood of political buy-in among stakeholders.

Management Information Systems

Compiling data to conform to performance measures and conducting the requisite analysis of the information will rely on the availability of computer platforms and software that align with the data collection protocols. In judging the efficiency of existing methods and the need for new processes, it is important to work directly with information technology staff at each stage of indicator development and implementation. It is also important to assess the ability of existing systems to generate reports and analyses that can be used to track trends and interpret data.

To minimize the staff hours and effort required to collect data, managers may want to look into "shortcuts," including the use of software for scanning and scoring, which eases survey administration and avoids the necessity of entering data by hand, and the use of personal digital assistants or laptop computers to enter data directly from the field into the database.

Although many public and private managers may not have access to sophisticated data systems—or may not even have direct authority over key data sets—this should not be an excuse for inaction. There are many less sophisticated, home-grown methods (e.g., using Excel spreadsheets) that can serve to launch a performance indicator system.

Cost of Survey Administration

Conducting face-to-face interviews with people with ID-DD is time and labor intensive. Several steps are involved in the process, including identifying potential interviewees, validating addresses and contact information, securing consent from the individual and the guardian, scheduling the interview, reviewing background and demographic information, and conducting the interview. In addition, interviewers must be recruited and trained.

There are various ways to control the costs of survey administration, and there are pros and cons of each. First, one can limit the sample size. This, however, may limit the manager's ability to confidently generalize the findings. In the NCI, for instance, each state is required to collect data on a randomly selected sample of 400 individuals, a sample size sufficient to generalize to the state but not to a substate level. Second, state or provider staff can be used to conduct interviews. This, however, requires a high level of vigilance to ensure that staff members do not have a direct connection to the individual (e.g., not on the case manager's active caseload) and that the interview does not take time away from other staff responsibilities. Third, volunteers, including families and self-advocates, can be used as interviewers. This option still has costs, because the recruitment and retention of volunteers is time consuming and travel must still be subsidized. Further, not paying people with ID-DD and/or families may be interpreted as exploitation and a lack of respect. Finally, costs can be reduced by staggering the data-collection cycles by either going to a survey every 2 years or conducting "rolling interviews" over a period of 2 years.

Stakeholder Support

Securing the support and "ownership" of stakeholders for the new performance measurement system is crucial and requires the careful and intentional involvement of people with ID-DD, their families, providers, and state staff—at each juncture of the process. Broad participation is necessary to ensure that the performance indicators reflect the interests and concerns of each constituency and to make sure that those responsible for generating and supporting data collection recognize the usefulness of the data. Finally, each constituency needs to be persuaded that the information generated from the data collection will provide it with information it needs to do its job, advocate, and assess quality.

Developing Norms and Benchmarks

In preparing to use performance indicators to assess the quality of a state, local, or provider program, managers need to answer the "compared to what?" question. There are various ways to secure appropriate comparative information.

First, data can be compared to existing data sets in other states or collected at the national level. For instance, to compare performance on work-related indicators, managers and other interested parties can review publications such as *State Data Reports* on employment of people with disabilities (Institute for Community Inclusion, 2005).

With respect to QOL indicators such as choice and empowerment, there are various state-supported consumer surveys, including the "Ask Me!" survey in Maryland (Bonham et al., 2004). An additional example is provided in Figure 7.1, which shows changes over 3 years in the proportion of individuals who reported in the NCI consumer survey that their case managers got them what they needed.

It is also possible to use benchmarks from the general population to determine the relative status of people with ID-DD in areas such as health. Figure 7.2 shows the comparison of the NCI multistate sample with the nationwide norm for attendance at the dentist within the past 6 months.

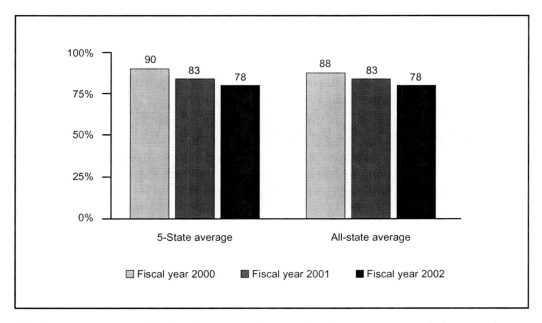

Figure 7.1. Percentage of individual respondents indicating case manager helps get what person needs.

Note. From *National Core Indicators: 5 Years of Performance Measurement,* by Human Services Research Institute and National Association of State Directors of Developmental Disabilities Services, 2003, Cambridge, MA, & Alexandria, VA. Used with permission.

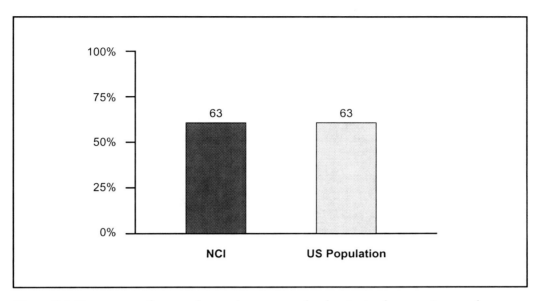

Figure 7.2. Percentage of respondents who went to the dentist in the past six months.

Note. National data from *Joint Canada/United States Survey of Health, 2002–2003,* by C. Sanmartin et al. 2003. Ottawa, ON: Statistics, Canada; Atlanta, GA: Centers for Disease Control and Prevention. NCI data from *National Core Indicators: 5 Years of Performance Measurement,* by Human Services Research Institute and National Association of State Directors of Developmental Disabilities Services, 2003, Cambridge, MA, & Alexandria, VA. Used with permission.

Comparing causes of death between people with cognitive disabilities and the general population is another powerful example of how performance data can be used. Table 7.3 shows the differences and similarities in cause of death over a 4-year period among people served by the Massachusetts Department of Mental Retardation, the national general population, and the state's general population.

Finally, performance comparisons can be made with baseline years. Figure 7.3 shows the aggregate percentage of families with children, families with adult family members at home, and families of people in residential supports that believe their case manager gets them what they and their family members need. The bars on the left represent a consistent 5-state sample; the bars on the right reflect all of the data collected during those same 3 years.

Summary

The development of performance indicators and measures should result in a rich base of information that can be used to judge the quality of services and supports provided to people with ID-DD. If indicators are developed correctly, the resulting data should

TABLE 7.3

Death Rate Among People With ID-DD in Massachusetts Compared With General Population

Rank	U.S. 2002	Massachusetts 2001	Massachusetts Dept. Mental Retardation 1999	Massachusetts Dept. Mental Retardation 2000	Massachusetts Dept. Mental Retardation 2001	Massachusetts Dept. Mental Retardation 2002
1	Heart disease	Heart disease	Heart disease	Heart disease	Heart disease	Heart disease
2	Cancer	Cancer	Pneumonia	Pneumonia	Aspiration pneumonia	Aspiration pneumonia
3	Stroke	Stroke	Chronic respiratory disease	Chronic respiratory disease	Cancer	Cancer and septicemia
4	Chronic respiratory disease	Chronic respiratory disease	Cancer	Cancer	Septicemia	Cardiac-pulminary arrest/seizure
5	Accidents	Influenza and pneumonia	Septicemia	Septicemia	Alzheimer's	Alzheimer's
6	Diabetes	Alzheimer's	Gastro-intestinal	Nephritis	Influenza and pneumonia	Chronic respiratory disease
7	Influenza and pneumonia	Unintentional injuries	Nephritis	Cardiac-pulminary arrest/seizure	Chronic respiratory disease	Influenza and pneumonia
8	Alzheimer's	Diabetes	Alzheimer's	Alzheimer's	Cardiac-pulminary arrest/seizure	Nephritis
9	Nephritis	Nephritis	Seizure-related	Stroke	Accidents	Stroke
10	Septicemia	Septicemia	Accidents	Gastro-intestinal	Stroke	Congenital defects

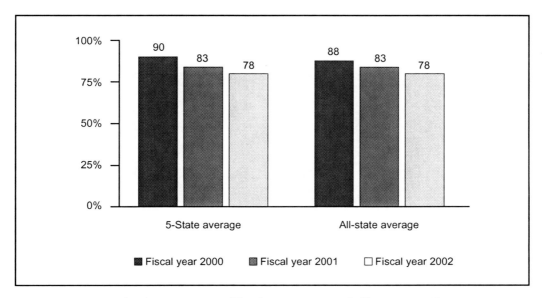

Figure 7.3. Longitudinal comparison of family perceptions of effectiveness of case managers.
Note. From *National Core Indicators: 5 Years of Performance Measurement,* by Human Services Research Institute and National Association of State Directors of Developmental Disabilities Services, 2003, Cambridge, MA, & Alexandria, VA. Reprinted with permission.

tell managers how well their programs and systems are delivering services consistent with their mission and meeting stakeholders' expectations for valued outcomes. To ensure that the resulting data is useful and comprehensive, managers should be prepared to follow through the project to its end.

The purpose of this chapter has been to provide the framework for developing performance indicators at the macro-system level. This framework involves the following sequential stages: selecting performance indicators, identifying and reviewing existing measures and data sources, conducting psychometric tests of the measures, designing data collection tools, selecting final measures, and developing norms and benchmarks.

Once these performance indicators are selected and validated, the emphasis within the system shifts to their use. That topic is the focus of the following chapter.

CHAPTER 8

How Do I Use Performance Indicator Data?

Introduction and Overview

Perhaps the most neglected aspect of performance measurement is the development of systematic mechanisms to use collected information to inform key constituencies, improve systems of supports, enhance the well-being of people with intellectual and developmental disabilities (ID-DD), and pursue quality improvement.

Public and private managers have not taken advantage of the collected data to mount systemic improvement for several reasons, one being that the data (e.g., personal outcomes, incident reporting, licensing, provider performance) is collected, managed, and housed in disparate agencies, a circumstance that has led to data "stovepipes." These stovepipes have prevented managers from developing an overall picture of the system and thus precluded looking at the entire system.

The parable of the blind men and the elephant is a good metaphor for these deconstructed viewpoints. This brief segment from John Godfrey Saxe's (1963) 19th-century poetic telling of an ancient fable highlights the problem:

> The first [blind man] approached the elephant, and, happening to fall,
> against his broad and sturdy side, at once began to bawl:
> "God bless me! but the elephant, is nothing but a wall!"

> The second feeling of the tusk, cried: "Ho! what have we here,
> so very round and smooth and sharp? To me 'tis mighty clear,
> this wonder of an elephant, is very like a spear!"

> The third approached the animal, and, happening to take,
> the squirming trunk within his hands, "I see," quoth he,
> "the elephant is very like a snake!"

The challenge for public managers is to find ways of viewing the entire system by integrating data systems and data analysis. Clearly this is a technical as well as a political challenge, given clashing jurisdictions and legacy database systems. However, in an increasingly complex and multifarious system of services and supports, state agencies and service providers can no longer afford to see only one part of the elephant.

The purpose of this chapter is to illustrate ways in which performance indicators can be used to facilitate compliance with state and federal requirements, to improve the understanding of the service system, and to enhance the adoption of more efficient and effective means of providing services and supports (i.e., to improve quality). The chapter concludes with a discussion of emerging practices and challenges in using quality of life (QOL)-related personal outcomes and performance indicators. A major challenge in that regard is for organizations and systems to reframe quality and rethink quality improvement, as discussed in the final section of the text.

Performance Data and Federal Requirements

New Evidence Requirements

As noted in chapter 6, the federal Centers for Medicare and Medicaid Services (CMS), through the adoption of more comprehensive expectations regarding quality assurance and quality improvement in Home and Community-Based Services (HCBS), have given states, localities, and providers a powerful impetus to collect, analyze, and apply valid and reliable performance data (U.S. Department of Health & Human Services, 2005). To be approved to provide HCBS waivers or to renew a current waiver, states will, by 2006, be required to develop a quality-management strategy that describes the performance data they collect, the ways in which they use the data to respond to individual issues, and the long-term use of the data for quality improvement. The evidence generated by the quality-management plan will be reviewed throughout the 5-year waiver cycle.

CMS will review data aggregated by the state and organized around the basic assurances and the Quality Framework shown previously in Figure 6.2. Each state will be required to align performance indicators with the quality components and describe the data collection protocols or discovery methods that will be used to generate evidence. Table 8.1 describes how some of the indicators and data collection sources from the National Core Indicators (NCI; Human Services Research Institute, 2003) can be applied to meet the new expectations of CMS.

Outlines of a Quality-Management Strategy

CMS is also interested in whether performance data is valid and reliable, and whether the information is used as part of an overall quality-management strategy that results in systemic improvement. In each new waiver and waiver renewal, states will be required to describe their quality-management plan. The following is a description of what

	Table 8.1 Crosswalk of National Core Indicators Data Sources to CMS Quality Framework		
CMS Quality Component	Performance Indicator		National Core Indicators Data Collection Element
1. Participant access	• Proportion of case managers who can communicate in other languages matches proportion of clients who prefer other languages.		Case management surveys
	• Proportion of eligible families that report having access to an adequate array of services and supports.		Family survey
2. Participant-centered service planning and delivery	• Proportion of case managers who support self-determination, choice, community integration, employment, and natural supports for individuals with developmental disabilities.		Case management survey
	• Individuals get the services they need.		Consumer survey
	• Proportion of families that report that their support plans include or reflect things that are important to them.		Family survey
3. Provider capacity and capabilities	• Proportion of families that report that service and support staff or providers are available and capable of meeting family needs.		Family survey
	• The crude separation rate, defined as the proportion of direct-contact staff separated in the past year.		Provider survey

(table continues)

TABLE 8.1 *(continued)*		
CMS Quality Component	**Performance Indicator Data Collection Element**	**National Core Indicators**
4. Participant safeguards	• Mortality rate of the served MR-DD population compared to the general area population, by age, by cause of death (natural or medico-legal), and by MR or DD diagnosis.	System data
	• Proportion of people who report that they feel safe in their home and neighborhood.	Consumer survey
5. Participant rights and responsibilities	• Proportion of people whose basic rights are respected by others.	Consumer survey
6. Participant outcomes and satisfaction	• Proportion of families that feel that services and supports have helped them to better care for their family member living at home.	Family surveys
	• Proportion of people who control their own budgets.	Consumer survey
7. System performance	• Proportion of individuals age 18 and over who receive services, compared to the estimated number of adults with a DD in a state's population.	Basic profile report

Note. CMS = U.S. Centers for Medicare and Medicaid Services. MR = mental retardation. DD = developmental disability(s).

CMS is anticipating with respect to quality management as laid out in the *Draft Application Version 3.1 for Use by States* (U.S. Department of Health & Human Services, 2005):

> A basic tenet of a QM [quality-management] strategy is that information is available on how well the system is performing and that it is used to improve

individual and system performance. This happens in two ways. First, through knowing what is happening to an individual participant and acting to remediate problems. Second, through determining how often a given event or process occurs across all participants and working to change behavior, policies or procedures to effect system improvement. To achieve systems change, data must be collected consistently across the program so that it can be counted in the aggregate. (p. 131)

Specifically, states must include the following as part of their quality-management strategy: the activities or processes related to discovery; the entities, organizations, and other stakeholders involved in the quality-management strategy including their roles and responsibilities; the sources of data used to measure whether the state meets the requirements and assurances; the frequency with which performance in each assurance is measured; and quality-management reports. These new preconditions for participation in the waiver will have ripple effects throughout the system of services and supports for people with ID-DD. First, they will require agreement throughout the system regarding what data will be collected. Further, managers and providers must assess the state of current data to determine whether it is sufficiently robust and consistent with the Quality Framework. One of the biggest hurdles will be identifying the technical resources necessary to store the data in a convenient fashion so it is available to individuals with monitoring responsibilities across the system (e.g., case managers, abuse and neglect investigators, licensers, etc.). Finally, public managers, policy makers, agencies, and stakeholders will need the support of data analysts and report creators who can match the needs of these decision makers with a reliable flow of trend information. This need highlights the importance of those three evaluation and support standards discussed at the end of chapter 6: product quality, process quality, and usefulness of the information.

This important initiative by CMS will further reinforce the importance of developing performance indicators and measures that both capture the mission of a state, locality, or provider and be aligned with federal monitoring imperatives. By leaving the details of the quality-management strategy to the state, CMS has allowed for the alignment of specific state circumstances with federal expectations.

Examples of Quality Improvement

NCI (Human Services Research Institute, 2003) have already had both long-range and immediate influences on the ways states monitor performance and use performance data to influence systemic change, to inform customers, and to help meet the new CMS requirements. In Massachusetts, NCI data are being used as the cornerstone for the state's strategic plan for the enhancement of services to people with intellectual disabilities. Additionally, Massachusetts, Washington, and Wyoming used NCI data as a means of introducing CMS monitors to the performance of their systems as part of their HCBS waiver reviews.

The Massachusetts Department of Mental Retardation (2004) also used performance data from NCI and state data sources as the cornerstone of their annual quality assurance report. Figure 8.1 shows a comparison (based on NCI consumer surveys) across settings and across a 2-year period of the proportion of people who report that they experience respectful interactions with staff.

In Pennsylvania the NCI data requirements and other state performance requirements have helped shape the design of a HCBS management information system. The system reflects the interaction between performance measures and the design of a business model for data warehousing, data reporting, and data access, and is critical to the ability of managers and others to use information systems to support their quality-management efforts.

Additionally the Pennsylvania system uses NCI information in conjunction with independent monitoring at the local level. It is also an integral part of their overall quality-management framework. Called Independent Monitoring for Quality (IM4Q), the effort is based in local county, nonprofit entities (e.g., local Arcs) and includes people with ID-DD and family members as surveyors. The following is a description of the purposes of the monitoring in Pennsylvania (Feinstein & Caruso 2003):

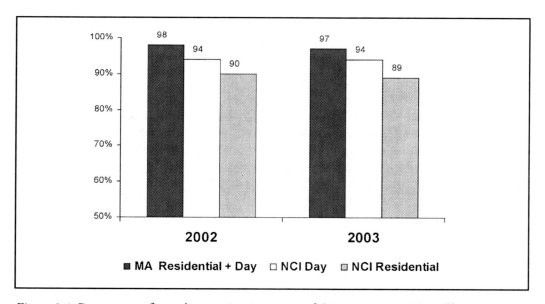

Figure 8.1. Percentage of people experiencing respectful interactions with staff.

Note. MA = Massachusetts. NCI = National Core Indicators. From *Quality Assurance Report for Fiscal Years 2002–2003.* Massachusetts Department of Mental Retardation, 2004. Boston. Reprinted with permission.

The IM4Q program is one part of a much larger effort by the Office of Mental Retardation [OMR] to provide continuous quality improvement in Pennsylvania. IM4Q is not meant to replace processes that now exist through OMR (e.g., licensing). IM4Q is unique in that people with disabilities, family members, and interested others, all of whom are without conflicts of interest from the mental retardation service/support/system, are the people interviewing people receiving services/support. This process provides an independent and external source of information which is not gathered by OMR, the county program, or provider systems. (pp. 184–185)

Many participating counties in Pennsylvania have adopted quality-management committees to explore the implications of the results of the consumer surveys in their service areas. Some of the initial findings include (Feinstein & Caruso, 2003):

- People should have a greater say over where they live and what they do during the day.

- People should have a more meaningful role in screening their potential roommates.

- A greater effort should be made to establish and use formal communications systems.

- Mail should not be read without permission.

- Friendships and family relationships should be supported with more opportunities to socialize.

- Complaint procedures should be as explicit as possible.

- Individuals should have their own set of keys.

These data have been presented by the steering committee to the state for their consideration. Activity has already commenced in several of the aforementioned areas where policy initiatives are required.

Other states have used the NCI performance data for a variety of other quality-management efforts. Arizona, for example, also uses NCI for Medicaid agency requirements; advertises reports in their newsletter; sends reports to all families who participated in the family survey; and shares their information with the legislature and governor. State staff have also used data to target improvements for women and to sharpen the understanding of families regarding their ability to choose their case managers. In Washington, the State Developmental Disabilities Council has appointed a special committee to review the state's family survey results and to make recommendations regarding changes in state policy.

Alabama uses the NCI consumer data as part of the data collection requirements in the *Wyatt v. Stickney* settlement. The court receives data on pre- and postlevels of satisfaction among individuals that leave Partlow Development Center to move into the community. The state DD agency, as a consequence of findings from the NCI consumer survey, identified the need for improvement in choice and decision making. As a consequence, the agency developed a 5-year plan to increase the numbers of person-centered planning facilitators and launched an initiative to provide Social Role Valorization (Wolfensberger, 1992) training to families.

To help state managers identify priorities for systemic improvement, Rhode Island has initiated a quality consortium to review statewide NCI and other data on systemic performance. An excerpt from the report presented to the consortium is included in

TABLE 8.2
Comparison of Consumer Outcomes: Rhode Island Quality Consortium

Data Source	Positive Trends	Areas for Improvement
Quality of Life Initiative (QLI)/National Core Indicators (NCI) (Fiscal Year 2000, Fiscal Year 2001) Consumer satisfaction	1. People are getting out for fun/social activities. 2. People like where they live. 3. People are making choices about everyday aspects of life. 4. Annual plans reflect what people really want. 5. Visitors provide great feedback on the interviews they have with people . . . visitors focus on strategies to communicate with people with limited communication skills.	1. Ongoing communication challenges of people. 2. Additional needs for support . . . tutorial, speech & language, mental health, employment, transportation, etc. 3. Loneliness . . . need for meeting new people for friendships. 4. More jobs for people. 5. People want to develop more relationships/ friendships with other individuals. 6. Capacity to visit more people on an annual basis. 7. Recruiting more visitors who are individuals with disabilities and people who are neighbors/ citizens who are not employed with a provider agency.

Note. From *The More We Know: Summary Information/Data From Various Initiatives, Projects, Reviews Relating to Systems,* by Rhode Island Division of Developmental Disabilities, 2003. Unpublished report prepared for the Rhode Island Consortium and based on 670 personal interviews.

Table 8.2 (Rhode Island Division of Developmental Disabilities, 2003). Based on these data, the consortium, comprised of a range of stakeholders, assessed the trends suggested by the data and chose three major priorities to work on: employment, relationships, and health and safety.

Rhode Island has also used data from the NCI to inform their risk management, incident prevention, and safety-planning process. Finally, results from NCI have led to concrete changes in licensing requirements for staff training, curriculum design, and professional development. Washington has used the data to revise their incident reporting and mortality data systems.

Several states have used the data to improve the responsiveness of the public system to consumers of services. In Vermont the state moved to improve accessibility of information on grievance systems when a significant number of consumers reported that they were unfamiliar with the process. At the Regional Center of Orange County (RCOC), California, program analysts noted that young families reported substantially less involvement than older families in their communities and were more dissatisfied with the information available to them regarding their service and support options. The center's staff took the following steps (Christianson, 2004):

- They created an early start survey to develop a deeper understanding of the needs of young families.

- They conducted staff training for typical childhood development for children 0 to 3 years and more than 3, to influence staff expectations.

- They provided more support and counseling to families of children under 18.

- They developed relationships with city recreation departments to facilitate more opportunities for community activities.

- They developed an RCOC newsletter, *Dialogue,* to provide a vehicle for the dissemination of information.

One State's Efforts

The state of Maine has integrated the performance data from NCI and other state data collection efforts into a comprehensive quality-management process that includes the following quality-improvement efforts (Gallivan, 2005):

- The Office of Quality Improvement (QI) conducts data collection using the NCI Consumer and Family Satisfaction Surveys.

- The Office of QI develops standard reports and summaries based on data.

- Standardized reports based on a core set of indicators are shared with the mental retardation program director.

- The mental retardation central management team reviews the reports to develop recommendations based on results of data.

- The mental retardation regional management teams review recommendations for development of implementation plan(s).

- The quality collaborative, composed of providers and self-advocates, review recommendations for an implementation plan.

- The mental retardation program director finalizes recommendations and the implementation plan.

- The mental retardation program director presents recommendation and the implementation plan to the executive management team.

- The state Mental Retardation Services Agency implements the plan.

- The Office of QI tracks recommendation and implementation.

One issue identified by the Maine Mental Retardation Services Agency through this quality-improvement process was the low numbers of individuals who reported having friends with whom they could talk. This finding identified a significant service or support need to state public managers and stakeholders. Results of addressing that need are summarized in Figure 8.2. As shown in the figure, while the number of people reporting they had friends went up from 2002 to 2003, the higher number (47.7%) is still relatively low (Gallivan, 2005).

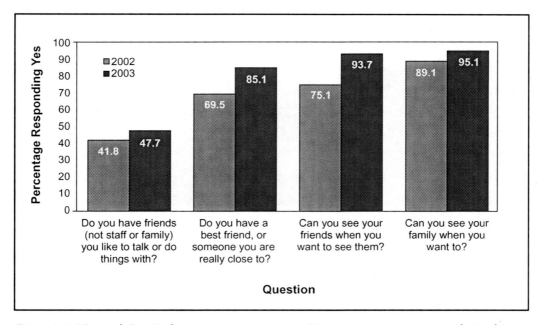

Figure 8.2. National Core Indicators consumers survey: Year-to-year comparison—relationships.

Note. From *National Care Indicators: 5 Years of Performance Measurement,* by Human Services Research Institute & National Association of State Directors of Developmental Disabilities Services, 2003, Cambridge, MA & Alexandria, VA. Used with permission.

In response to these data, the Office of QI has chosen to target *relationships,* setting the following goal for the ensuing round of data collection: "To increase the percentage of individuals reporting that they 'have friends that are not staff or family' by 5% based on the results of the National Core Indicators Consumer Survey by June 2005" (Gallivan, 2005).

A second issue was also identified through Maine's quality-improvement process and through an analysis of family survey data for the state compared to the national norms. The results showed that family members in Maine had lower than average positive response rates when queried about the feelings of choice and control regarding the configuration and type of services and supports for their family member with a disability. As a consequence, the state has instituted a number of changes including the development of an Independence Plus waiver, expansion of case management for families, and the preparation of brochures and a Web site for families seeking information on available services.

This case example underscores some basic principles that should govern quality improvement in public systems as well as in the private sector. First and foremost, the quality-improvement effort should be governed by the mission and values of the organization or agency. Second, data collection should be tailored to performance measures that square with the aspirations envisioned in the mission. Third, the information should be acted upon in a systematic fashion. Fourth, the quality-improvement effort should lead to concrete changes in practices and policies. Finally, the results of changes should be evaluated to make sure that the intervention had the hoped-for impact.

Using Performance Indicator Data: Emerging Practices and Challenges

Information for Consumers and Families

Provider Profiles
One of the next frontiers in the use of performance indicators is making outcome information available by individual provider. This would give individuals and families criteria they can use to make decisions regarding services and supports to meet their needs (Keith & Bonham, 2005). Examples were discussed earlier in reference to Nebraska (Ferdinand & Smith, 2002) and Maryland (Bonham et al., 2004). The development of such profiles, however, is still in the embryonic stage in most states. A few states (e.g., CT & WY) place the results of licensing reviews on their Web sites, but such efforts are minimal.

There are several reasons why the routine publication of provider profiles is still not widely employed. First, many states still maintain data in isolated "silos" that cannot be integrated easily. Although it is time consuming and expensive to develop a picture of a particular provider using incident, licensing, case-management, and other data, many states are beginning to integrate these data for their own quality assurance purposes. For example, accreditation staff in Ohio have relevant incident data when they do their yearly county monitoring, and Tennessee quality monitors review all relevant provider data before making their yearly review.

The second constraint is the validity and robustness of the performance indicator data used. Data used to support public reviews of providers will have to be viewed as objective by providers before they will grant the political support for such an initiative. The pressure to ensure that the data are accurate becomes even more profound when such data are used to determine funding levels. For example, the state of Georgia had to back down from a decision to use QOL data as a partial determinant of reimbursement, because the providers immediately attacked both the instrument and the administration.

A further issue involves the complexity of the current system of services and supports in many states. Most people now receive services from a range of providers, including residential supports, job supports, habilitation supports, and service brokerage. How can the accomplishment of positive or negative outcomes be attributed to one specific provider, when the individual has experiences with multiple interventions?

Finally, some state officials argue that making performance data available by provider is not a priority in areas where there are no choices of providers, particularly in rural areas or geographic areas where one provider dominates. Although this may be a valid concern, it is seemingly trumped by the need of individuals and families to know how their providers are performing.

Going forward, the release of provider-specific information will be accomplished when there is trust in the data collected and there is a collaboration and effort among state managers, providers, and individuals and families regarding what outcomes are most important, how the information is disseminated, and how the release of outcome data contributes to the system's overall improvement.

State Performance Data on Web Sites

Another important emerging practice involves the placement, on a regular basis, of performance results on state Web sites. Some states have begun to use their Web sites as a way of communicating their results with the public. For example, both Vermont (2005) and Massachusetts (2004) have used the Web to share their annual performance results.

Alignment With Other Sources of Information

To date, most of the quality-improvement efforts that rely on performance indicators have focused on data from the developmental disabilities system. Breaking down the silos within the system is important, but there are also possible insights that can be gleaned from other relevant information systems. One source of data on services outside of the disability system is Medicaid claims data. The virtue of using this data source is that it encompasses a broad range of health care services, including medications, and can be used to augment analyses of quality, cost, and access. For example, the Maine Mental Retardation Agency used Medicaid claims data to track the use of psychotropic medications to elderly individuals on the state's Eldercare waiver. The analysis involved aligning psychotropic drug use among waiver recipients with a formula constructed to identify potentially inappropriate medications for seniors. A recent presentation (Payne, 2005) summarized initial results regarding measuring and monitoring special quality problems:

- Many individuals in the sample had multiple prescribers.

- Many individuals were taking multiple medications.

- Some of the potential medication-related problems included overdose, death, frequent falls, frequent physician visits, hospital stays, and long-term care admissions.

- Individuals in the sample had multiple medical and mental health conditions.

- A number of individuals had chronic pain.

- There were many incidences of polypharmacy and potential drug interactions.

The challenges involved in using Medicaid data for purposes such as those described above include the fact that Medicaid data do not include any functional-level data. Further, to link Medicaid and waiver data requires a fair amount of technical skill and substantial computing power.

Public and private managers should also explore other sources of information that can be aligned with quality data from the ID-DD system. For instance, census data can be a valuable tool for assessing equity across the system. By comparing the numbers of individuals served from various ethnic and racial minorities with the total numbers of such individuals in the total population, public managers can determine whether there is equal access in the system. Regional calculations can also be made to determine whether there is equity across geographic areas.

The *Supports Intensity Scale* (Thompson et al., 2004) is another recent source of information that can play a potentially valuable role in understanding the allocation of resources across the system. The scale, which assesses the needs for supports among people with intellectual disabilities in a range of domains, can be aggregated and matched with services provided. This will allow managers at the state and provider level to identify the extent to which individuals are underserved or overserved—findings that help to realign resources in a more cost effective fashion.

Empowerment of Individuals and Families in the Process
It will be important for public and private managers to capitalize on the possibilities that performance indicator data provide for enhancing the participation of individuals and families in the quality assurance and quality-improvement process. Such

involvement can be through the collection of information as well as through the analysis of information. In Pennsylvania (e.g., Feinstein & Caruso, 2003) individuals and families participate in the collection of information regarding the achievement of valued outcomes. In Kentucky people with ID-DD form the teams that carry out the NCI surveys.

The other, and equally important, role played by individuals and families is as members of quality-improvement committees. The perspective of self-advocates and families is crucial to the assessment of the results of performance measurements. Many states, including Pennsylvania, Massachusetts, and Tennessee, are beginning to include these stakeholders in their quality-improvement process.

Summary

In moving forward, public and private managers need to find ways of turning the information they currently collect into an integrated performance assessment platform that allows them to look at outcomes from multiple perspectives and in ways that help them assess whether positive outcomes are being achieved. The process, to be successful, must be inclusive and transparent. Without information about all facets of the service delivery enterprise and the right eyes to view it, the elephant will continue to be viewed by blinkered observers who have no sense of the overall skeleton that gives it purpose.

In addition, public and private managers need to think differently about quality assurance and quality improvement. In the final section of the book we discuss how the QOL concept as reflected in personal outcomes and performance indicators requires people to reframe quality and rethink quality improvement. In that process we propose that quality assurance precedes quality improvement, and that the concept of quality assurance, which is in a state of transition, is about remediation and basic assurances. We propose further that the major purpose of quality improvement is to reduce the discrepancy between desired personal outcomes and objective conditions within the person's community. This quality-improvement imperative is accomplished through the use of information, data, and feedback (or some combination thereof) to enhance policy, practices, training, technical assistance, and other organizational and systems-level supports.

PART 4

Quality of Life for People With Intellectual and Other Developmental Disabilities: Going Forward

Thus far in the text, we have addressed four of the book's five objectives:

- To rethink what is meant by quality of life and how the quality of life (QOL) concept has become a change agent. In that regard, we linked various developments in the field of intellectual and developmental disabilities (ID-DD) to the evolution of the QOL concept and its use.

- To synthesize current research and literature in the area of quality of life and its measurement and discuss how the concept has influenced management strategies, organizational design, systems change, and leadership. As we will discuss in chapter 9, we need to do this within the context of community networks of resources and supports.

- To provide examples of how the QOL concept can be operationalized, measured, and applied at the individual, organizational, and systems level. In this process, we (a) presented a set of criteria and guidelines regarding its conceptualization, measurement, and application, and (b) discussed how QOL-related information can be integrated at the individual, organizational, and systems level.

- To show how QOL-related information can be used in an intentional way to enhance personal outcomes. In the process, we illustrated several factors that are influencing how we do business and how we measure performance. Chief among these are (a) basing services on person-centered supports and self-determination, (b) focusing on personal outcomes in addition to quality processes, (c) recognizing the changes in experiences

and expectations of consumers and families, (d) moving away from prescriptive standards, (e) emphasizing quality improvement, and (f) involving consumers in the design,
delivery, and evaluation of services and supports.

In the process of meeting these four objectives, we discussed factors related to the
conceptualization, measurement, and application of the QOL concept. These factors
lead directly to our discussion in the final section of the text of (a) enhancing people's
quality of life by reframing quality, rethinking quality improvement, overcoming
challenges to all stakeholders as they improve their lives, and (b) embracing the
opportunities provided by the QOL concept and its application to people with ID-
DD across individuals, organizations, communities, and systems.

In review of the *QOL concept,* as discussed throughout the text, quality of life is a
multidimensional phenomenon composed of core QOL domains and indicators
(see Tables 2.3–2.7). Fundamental principles regarding its conceptualization are that
quality of life is influenced by personal and environmental factors and their interaction;
has the same components for all people; has both subjective and objective
components; and is enhanced by self-determination, resources, purpose in life, and a
sense of belonging.

Three key points about *QOL measurement* were made throughout the preceding
eight chapters. First, measurement involves the assessment of QOL indicators reflective
of QOL domains that are based on a validated QOL model. Second, QOL
measurement is a two-component process that involves: (a) an in-person interview to
determine personal outcomes, and (b) then placing the person within the context of
objective conditions within his or her community to determine how well the outcomes
are being met. As we discuss more fully in chapter 9, the purpose of quality
improvement is to bring the two (i.e., the desires and the realities) closer together.
Third, QOL measurement is guided by four principles, that it (a) involves the degree
to which people have life experiences that they value, (b) reflects the domains that
contribute to a full and interconnected life, (c) considers the contexts of physical,
social, and cultural environments that are important to people, and (d) includes
measures of experiences both common to all people and those unique to individuals.

The *application of the QOL concept* across the micro, meso, and macro systems is
occurring within major changes in social policy and organizational practices. Chief
among these are (Schalock & Luckasson, 2005): (a) a transformed vision of what
constitutes the life possibilities of people with ID-DD, including an emphasis on self-
determination, community inclusion, equity, and human potential; (b) an ecological
conception of disability that focuses on the person and the environment; (c) the
development of community-based options and support systems; (d) the
implementation of service options, including the direct purchase of services and
supports; (e) the use of the QOL concept as the basis for best practices; (f) the
emergence of the reform movement with its emphasis on measurability, reportability,

and accountability; and (g) the use of QOL-related outcome information for multiple purposes including the provision of information, improving services and supports, and guiding the change process.

Collectively, these changes influence the rationale for organizational and systems-level performance indicators that reflect social policy that emphasize personal outcomes and the increasing need for accountability and quality improvement.

Throughout the integration of these factors related to the conceptualization, measurement, and application of the QOL concept to people with ID-DD, we have stressed that the large-scale adoption of a person-centered approach to basic assurances and quality of life and its application requires a data-based quality model that results in the development of new and improved assessment methodologies grounded in person-centered assurances and QOL principles. Material presented in the preceding eight chapters provides the framework for such a data-driven QOL model.

The full implementation of that QOL system involves not just the implementation of those conceptualization, measurement, and application factors mentioned above; it also includes implementing our fifth objective: to move beyond traditional terms and concepts, such as standards, program-specific requirements, process measurement, and quality as compliance, to a QOL focus with its emphasis on the achievement of personal outcomes. Basic to this achievement is a quality-improvement process that emphasizes the achievement of personal outcomes by reducing the discrepancy between the person's desired personal outcomes and objective conditions within his or her community. As we discuss in the following two chapters, this process requires that all stakeholders: (a) reframe quality and rethink quality improvement (chap. 9), and (b) address, as we do in chapter 10, six emerging challenges and opportunities related to quality of life as a change agent, QOL assessment and feedback as an integral part of how organizations and systems operate, consumers as key players, organizations redefining their roles, new management strategies, and quality improvement as a continuous process.

In reading this final section of the text, the reader will appreciate again the evolutionary nature of the QOL concept. As discussed in chapter 1, historically the QOL concept was used primarily as a sensitizing notion that gave us reference and guidance as to what is valued and desired from the individual's perspective. As reflected in the text so far, its role has expanded to include: (a) a conceptual framework for assessing personal outcomes, (b) a social construct that guides quality-improvement strategies, (c) a criterion for assessing the effectiveness of those strategies, and (d) the framework for an evidence-based quality-improvement model. These changes reflect clearly that the QOL concept has become an agent for social change that at its core makes us think differently about people with ID-DD and how we might bring about change at the organizational, community, and systems level to enhance their personal outcomes.

CHAPTER 9

Reframing Quality and Rethinking Quality Improvement

Introduction and Overview

Our definitions, indicators, and outcomes, as well as our methods of measuring and evaluating quality, are grounded in tradition and past practice. Both our values and systems of metrics are historically based. These values, once accepted and grounded in individual and organizational behavior, are difficult to change. Why? Because, in general, the capability and function of current systems, designed decades ago, determine what and how we measure. Thus we attempt to move forward using systems based on traditional values and legacy information.

Sam Walter Foss captured this reality in his hundred-year-old poem "The Calf-Path":

One day, through the primeval wood,
A calf walked home, as good calves should;
But made a trail all bent askew,
A crooked trail, as all calves do.

Since then three hundred years have fled,
And, I infer, the calf is dead.
But still he left behind his trail,
And thereby hangs my moral tale.

The trail was taken up next day
By a lone dog that passed that way;
And then a wise bellwether sheep
Pursued the trail o'er vale and steep,
And drew the flock behind him, too,
As good bellwethers always do.

And from that day, o'er hill and glade,
Through those old woods a path was made,
And many men wound in and out,
And dodged and turned and bent about,
And uttered words of righteous wrath
Because 'twas such a crooked path;
But still they followed—do not laugh—
The first migrations of that calf,
And through this winding wood-way stalked.
Because he wobbled when he walked.

This forest path became a lane,
That bent, and turned, and turned again.
This crooked lane became a road,
Where many a poor horse with his load
Toiled on beneath the burning sun,
And traveled some three miles in one.
And thus a century and a half
They trod the footsteps of that calf.

The years passed on in swiftness fleet.
The road became a village street,
And this, before men were aware,
A city's crowded thoroughfare,
And soon the central street was this
Of a renowned metropolis;
And men two centuries and a half
Trod in the footsteps of that calf.

Each day a hundred thousand rout
Followed that zigzag calf about,
And o'er his crooked journey went
The traffic of a continent.
A hundred thousand men were led
By one calf near three centuries dead.
They follow still his crooked way,
And lose one hundred years a day,
For thus such reverence is lent
To well-established precedent.

A moral lesson this might teach
Were I ordained and called to preach;
For men are prone to go it blind

Along the calf-paths of the mind,
And work away from sun to sun
To do what other men have done.
They follow in the beaten track,
And out and in, and forth and back,
And still their devious course pursue,
To keep the path that others do.

They keep the path a sacred groove,
Along which all their lives they move;
But how the wise old wood-gods laugh,
Who saw the first primeval calf!
Ah, many things this tale might teach—
But I am not ordained to preach.

Changing these calf-paths of our individual and collective thinking is a continual challenge. Albert Einstein noted that we can never solve problems unless we rise above the level of awareness that created the problem. He also concluded that our theories determine what we measure. Kuhn (1961) defined scientific paradigms as the constellation of shared values, concepts, and techniques. He noted that communities identified and examined legitimate problems and solutions only within the identified paradigm. He also drew attention to the importance of infrequent "paradigm shifts," discontinuous and revolutionary breaks with tradition.

Senge (1990) offered the term "mental models" to describe the simple generalizations or complex theories that "shape how we act" (p. 175). He noted the power of mental models in governing thinking and behavior with reference to the fable "The Emperor's New Clothes," where people's mental models prevented them from seeing the emperor's nakedness.

Management and organizational commentators have noted the difficulty of using old thinking, paradigms, frames, and mental models to solve new problems. Stacey (1992) remarked that old maps are useless in new terrain, and Vail (1993) drew attention to the futility of using a topographical map in the midst of an earthquake. Langer (1997) indicated that it is "easier to learn something the first time than it is to unlearn it and then to learn it differently" (p. 85). Finally, over the past quarter century, Bolman and Deal (2003) have borrowed from clinical psychology and psychiatry the metaphor and methodology of "reframing" and offered guidance on how to change our thinking about organizations. Thus in this chapter *we challenge the reader to reframe quality and rethink quality improvement.*

Six Mental Models

Our definitions and measurement of quality—quality assurance, quality of service, and quality of life—have evolved, and continue to evolve, from generally accepted paradigms, frames, or mental models. But each of these paradigms has in turn generated its own antithesis. The result is that our dialogue on reframing quality is engulfed in the tension, ambiguity, and paradox of both declining and emerging frames, or what we will refer to as mental models. Our discussion of reframing quality and rethinking quality improvement begins with a summary of six dualities or mental models: (a) reductionism versus systems thinking, (b) mechanistic versus organic organizations, (c) analysis versus synthesis, (d) planned versus self-organizing emergent systems, (e) thinking versus doing, and (f) tacit versus implicit knowledge. Each of these models affects how we approach the conceptualization, measurement, and application of the QOL concept.

Reductionism Versus Systems Thinking

Reductionism is often associated with the scientific method. Reductionism emphasizes that a complex phenomenon can best be understood by examining smaller, more basic aspects of the phenomenon (Capra, 1982). Chambers (1997) defined reductionism as "reducing the complex and varied to the simple and standard" (p. 42), and he noted that it focuses on parts rather than the whole. Senge (1990) voiced a similar concern when he defined reductionism as the "pursuit of simple answers to complex problems" (p. 175). Examples of reductionism abound. Biochemistry is based on the premise that the properties and functions of organisms can be explained in terms of the laws of chemistry and physics. The fragmentation of business enterprises into engineering, manufacturing, finance, and marketing illustrates the functionality of reductionism. The proponents of Total Quality Management (TQM) and Continuous Quality Improvement (CQI) referred to this phenomenon as "silo" management.

The field of ID-DD has often used reductionism to manage the complex. IQ tests, behavior modification, diagnostic labels, typologies, singular classification systems, quality assurance checklists, and satisfaction surveys offer quick and simple substitutes for complex and ambiguous situations.

Systems thinking evolved in the 1940s in response to the reductionism in science. Recognizing the distinction between substance and structure (i.e., variables) and form (i.e., patterns and relationships among the variables), systems theory emphasized the mapping and understanding of patterns. Systems thinking shifts attention from the "things" of knowledge to a focus on relationships (Capra, 1996, 2002; Senge, 1990; Wheatley, 1994).

Instead of isolating elements under observation, systems theory emphasizes the relationship between and among the parts that, taken together, make up the whole phenomenon. Researchers have commented on the connection between general systems theory and quantum theory and the "new physics" (Capra, 1996, 2002; Flynn, 2003; Waldrop, 1992; Wheatley, 1994, 1996). Capra (2002) noted, for example, the interconnected web of relations throughout modern science, and Wheatley (1994) declared that the "unseen connections between what were previously thought to be separate entities are the fundamental elements of all creation" (p. 10).

Systems theory provides an integrated and connected view of organizations and performance. It focuses attention on connections between and among entities and events or conditions that we might otherwise view as independent. A systems approach helps us understand the complexity of, and ambiguous connections between and among, all the supports and services offered to people with ID-DD. We can begin to understand that basic assurances in health, safety, and human security are connected to community, choice, and friendships. As shown in Figure 9.1, organizational functions are connected, and changes in one system influence the other components.

Mechanistic Versus Organic Organizations

The mechanistic-organic dichotomy describes characteristics of organizations and systems. Mechanistic models are based on industrial-era organization and are characterized by regulation, rules, policy and procedure, centralization, and a clear hierarchy of authority (Burns & Stalker, 1961). Mechanistic systems typically exist in situations that are large-scale, that emphasize efficiency, and that involve routine and repetitive technology. The goal of mechanistic systems is to eliminate surprise and uncertainty. Mintzberg (1989) noted that in mechanistic systems rules and regulations

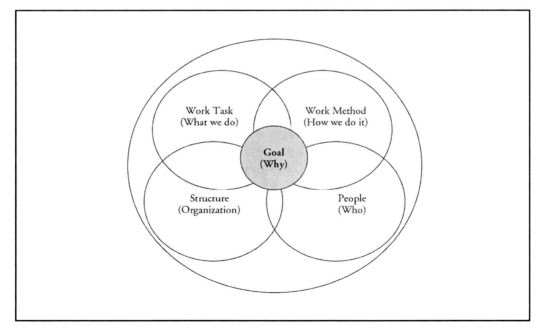

Figure 9.1. Integrated systems thinking.

permeate the system, and power rests at the top. He observed that such organizations operate smoothly and without interruption, and that control is an obsession.

In contrast, organic control models, which include feedback, coordination, priority setting, and communication patterns, exist in changing environments where work tasks are not repetitive and routine. Decentralized structures and feedback are based on values, norms, and traditions rather than rules alone. Decision making includes trial and error, learning through doing, and the organization tolerates more conflict between units. Organic models in human services decentralize decision-making responsibility, increase the autonomy and power of people receiving services, and decrease the role and power of professionals and bureaucrats. Organic models change and evolve in response to their environment.

Many community systems and services still maintain the mechanistic characteristics of the older state institutions from which they evolved in terms of rules, regulation, workforce management and supervision, and hierarchy and control. In fact, even in progressive organizations and systems, the mechanistic versus organic continuum is not absolute. Organizations generally display elements of both types of systems. For example, while we promote the development of organic, flexible systems of support for people, we also demand mechanistic controls over the basic assurances of health, safety, and human security.

In addition, some stakeholders remain ambivalent about the organic model. We recognize that mechanistic systems don't work, because they can't anticipate the range of individual needs, preferences, and behavior. Plans are unable to anticipate the diversity or intensity of unanticipated situations. Organic systems evolve and change in response to the individual and changing environments. Nonetheless, the concerns that Kelly (1995) identified about organic systems, "decentralized, self-making systems" (p. 194), are major continuing concerns for families, public officials, and support providers: You can't understand them; you have less control; they don't optimize well.

Analysis Versus Synthesis
An analytic approach to problem solving is based on the premise that we understand phenomenon best when we break them down into progressively smaller units of discovery. We focus attention on the individual units of inquiry. In many instances we narrow our analysis to what has been measured and captured in legacy data bases (Chambers, 1997). In contrast, synthesis proceeds by bringing individual components together so we can better understand the larger phenomenon. Synthesis focuses on the relationships between and among the parts, not on the isolated parts themselves (Capra, 1996).

Senge (1990) pointed to the difference between detailed and dynamic complexity. Detailed complexity concerns itself with as many variables (parts) in the situation as possible. In contrast, synthesis depends on dynamic complexity where the relationships between and among parts are subtle and often ambiguous. Senge noted that "complex arrays of details can actually distract us from seeing patterns and major interrelationships" (p. 72). He warned us against devising solutions that involved detailed complexity for problems that, rather, demanded solutions involving synthesis and a better understanding of dynamic complexity. This observation is similar to that of Georgia O'Keefe (1976), who noted that "Nothing is less real than realism. Details are confusing. It's only by selection, by elimination, by emphasis that we get the real meaning of things" (p. 87).

Kelly (1995) made a similar point in retelling the narrative about the steel industry's pre-1950 attempts to roll sheet metal to a uniform thickness. They

> discovered about a half-dozen factors that affected the thickness of the steel grinding out of the rolling mill—such as the speed of the rollers, temperature of the steel, and the traction of the sheets—and spent years strenuously perfecting the regulation of each of them. . . . To no avail. . . . The control of one factor would unintentionally disrupt the other factors. Slowing the speed would raise the temperature; lowering the temperature would raise the traction; increasing traction lowers speed. Everything was influencing everything else. (p. 120)

Most of our challenges in human services and ID-DD require us to apply synthesis and dynamic complexity. We need to understand the relationships between naturally emerging support networks and basic safety and well-being; determine the relationships between personal quality of life, formal support systems, informal organic networks and community indicators that influence quality; and have fewer details and more synthesis and understanding.

Planned Versus Self-Organizing Emergent Systems
The planning model is a reasonable response to attempted change. The link between cause and effect and our ability to predict and plan for consequences provides an indicator of our individual, social, and cultural development. Advances in science and technology have demonstrated the contributions of the planning model: Planning in the personal, family, business, or public administration context enables us to anticipate and sequence events and variables. But our traditional planning models are displaying limits.

Successful planning requires the requisite amount of data and information. Insufficient knowledge limits our planning ability. Even with adequate information, we often fail to anticipate the secondary and tertiary consequences of our actions. Our analytical and reductionist models fail to anticipate consequences outside our immediate systems of concern. Hence technological solutions to one problem generate a second set of problems. Tenner (1996) captured this phenomenon in the title *Why Things Bite Back: Technology and the Revenge of Unintended Consequences.*

More important, however, planning models, even with sufficient information, have limited usefulness. Planning models emphasize data, analysis, and prediction. We believe that we can anticipate, define, and measure a future phenomenon. The metaphor of an engineering model describes our planning efforts. But engineering models work best in static, controlled (i.e., mechanistic) systems. We can design bridges between two points. When neither point can be defined, however, nor the range of variation established, linear planning models fail us. Waldrop (1992) noted that "top-down systems are forever running into combinations of events they don't know how to handle" (p. 279).

Recent advances in the physical and social sciences suggest new alternatives for looking at change. "Self-organizing" systems and "emergence" emphasize network and web relationships among systems, events, and variables (Capra, 1996; Helgesen, 1995). Self-organizing systems shape our physical and social world. They demonstrate that new structures, patterns, and properties can emerge without being planned or externally imposed. Coordination and feedback generally exist throughout the system and are not planned or imposed from a central hierarchy. Self-organizing systems develop through emergence. They organize in ways that we cannot predict. In contrast to the engineering metaphor, emergence suggests a model of "biological adaptation." Wheatley and Kellner-Rogers (1996) summarized the concept this way:

> An emergent world asks us to stand in a different place. We can no longer stand at the end of something we visualize in detail and plan backwards from that future. Instead we must stand at the beginning, clear in our intent, with a willingness to be involved in discovery. The world asks that we focus less on how we can coerce something to make it conform to our designs and focus more on how we can engage with one another, how we can enter into the experience and notice that come forth. It asks that we participate more than plan. (p. 73)

Leadership responsibilities in the field of human services and ID-DD plunge us into a necessary tension. We must plan and provide accountability, but at the same time we must recognize the importance of self-organizing and emergent systems for people with disabilities and those who support them. We have long recognized the constraints imposed on the formation of future visions by labels and an overemphasis on weaknesses. Plans limit our thinking in the same way. Yet we continue to "plan" our way to resource allocation, accountability, and goal attainment even though we recognize that the people's possibilities for the future have not yet emerged. We also know that no amount of planning and engineering necessarily results in friendships, support networks, or social capital.

Maybe we can plan to optimize current knowledge and resources, but we must then encourage the processes and relationships of self-organization and emergence. Maybe we can plan for contingencies and safety-net back-ups when emergence threatens health and safety. Maybe planning and emergence can blend into a realized strategy.

Thinking Versus Doing

Organizational systems with a mechanistic orientation generally separate the functions of "learning" and "doing." Helgesen (1995) referred to the distinction as one between conception and execution. Frederick Taylor, the leader of the scientific management revolution in the early 1900s, promoted "specialization" and used scientific data to separate the planning (i.e., thinking) from the work performance (i.e., doing). Taylor's work spread worldwide and influenced organizational design for the next century. Top management was responsible to strategic management; middle management standardized the operating policy and procedures; and bottom-level workers performed the designated tasks (Savage, 1996).

The separation results in two problems. First, the "thinkers" become dependent upon data and information that is increasingly filtered as it moves to the top of the hierarchy. Important information becomes synonymous with codification, quantitative data, and analysis. Soft information about people, values, meaning, and synthesis filters out as it travels across organizations and upward through hierarchies. Thinking and planning are removed from the field of implementation, application, and impact of work methods. The second problem is that top managers learn from filtered data rather than from doing.

Recent trends in the academic research, clinical psychology, quality management, organizational design, and new science are leading toward (a) reintegrating thinking and doing (Schein, 1992); (b) reflecting on our actions (Maturana & Varela, 1992; Piaget, 1971); and (c) coordinating our actions and activities (Sandow & Allen, 2004). Action research, which is reflective of these trends and is also an essential part of reframing quality, is based on a model of learning from doing and then acting based on that knowledge; doing and our subsequent actions do not result from planning alone. As discussed by Sandow and Allen (2004) and Wheatley (1994), abstract planning divorced from action becomes a cerebral activity of conjuring up a world that does not exist, whereas learning and reflection resulting from doing represents a scientific process for acquiring dynamic knowledge.

This reintegration of doing and thinking is vital for the field of human services and ID-DD, because we can't begin to define either a final goal or environment for people until we give them the opportunity to act and learn in that environment. New environments and experiences provide the opportunities to learn from doing. This concept applies not only to people receiving services and supports, but also directly addresses organizations and their employees (Helgesen, 1995). Sandow and Allen (2004) concluded, "We have discovered the most profound knowledge of collaboration emerges in the doing—that is, as we work and reflect on our work with others" (p. 10).

Tacit Versus Explicit Knowledge

The linkage of learning from doing to all members of the organization highlights the importance of integrating tacit and explicit knowledge (Nonaka & Takeuchi, 1995; Von Krough, Ichije, & Nonaka, 2000). Explicit information is easily shared and transferred. It can be reproduced and communicated in reports and narratives as well as in checklists, databases, journal articles, and book chapters.

In contrast, tacit knowledge is often referred to as "soft" information. Tacit knowledge refers to the skills, information, and ways of working that we accumulate over years. In addition, tacit knowledge includes feelings about values, norms, and expectations. These are attitudes that we find almost impossible to convey in an organization's orientation session, mission statement, or employee handbook. Staff acquires this knowledge through "doing" or "talking with" the right people.

We sometimes refer to tacit knowledge as intuitive. This tacit knowledge is processed and internalized by the knower over long periods of time. Davenport and Prusak (1998) described tacit knowledge as rich, complex, and undocumented as well as difficult to teach, articulate, or observe. Above all, they noted that it is almost impossible to reproduce in a document or database. "The codification process for the richest tacit knowledge in organizations is generally limited to locating someone with the knowledge, pointing the seeker to it, and encouraging them to interact" (p. 71).

Tacit information is not found in books, reports, or databases. Rather, it is oral. It is grounded in people's values, norms, and expectations about the work environment, their responsibilities, and their co-workers. People create and share tacit information while working together and discussing their work around the water cooler or at the coffeehouse. This kind of information spreads when people meet and tell stories (Stone, 1996). Deal and Kennedy (1999) indicated that "storytelling is one of the most powerful ways to convey information and shape behavior" (p. 9). Tacit information is conveyed at bus stops, in restaurants, backyards, and libraries. People with ID-DD, their families, friends, and supporters depend on tacit information.

Tacit information is difficult to transfer, because it is difficult to document or communicate; it is often too subtle and complex for normal language and text. However, the most important factor influencing the communication of tacit information may be trust (Bruhn, 2001; Seligman, 1997). People evaluate information based on their perception of the people providing the information. Water cooler dialogue diminishes in the presence of people who don't merit our full trust and confidence. Thus the presence of tacit knowledge presents us with three challenges:

1. Recognize the value of stories, music, art, and other media that encourage people to acquire and transfer tacit information.

2. Recognize that the acquisition and transfer of tacit knowledge depends on trust. Trust is the silent connector in social networks. When people listen to learn and learn to listen to others, they begin to build shared meaning that is critical for

collaboration and the flow of knowledge (Sandow & Allen, 2004). Neither sharing, knowledge transfer, nor social networks can exist without trust.

3. Make tacit knowledge explicit and explicit knowledge tacit by internalizing values and beliefs; otherwise it cannot be widely shared, examined, or improved. Davenport and Prusak (1998) concluded that "It's a never ending cycle: Identifying tacit information; making it explicit so that it can be formalized, captured and leveraged; encouraging the new knowledge to soak in and become tacit" (p. 74).

Thus reframing quality and rethinking quality improvement are not just about understanding the conceptualization, measurement, and application of the QOL concept. As important as this understanding is, enhancing the quality of life of people with ID-DD requires different mental models than the ones used in the previous approaches to individuals, organizations, and systems. As just discussed, this new mental model is characterized by the six elements summarized in Table 9.1.

Three Organizing Principles

These six elements not only characterize our reframing of quality and rethinking quality improvement, they also provide the basis for three organizing principles: social

---

TABLE 9.1
Strategies Characterizing a "Reframing Quality" and "Rethinking Quality Improvement" Mental Model

---

1. Embrace systems theory that provides an integrated and connected view of organizations and performance.

2. Employ an organic model in human services that stresses decentralized decision-making responsibility, increased autonomy and power of people receiving services, and decreased role and power of professionals and bureaucrats.

3. Focus on a synthesis approach that brings together individual components to better understand the larger phenomenon.

4. Develop self-organizing systems that emphasize network and web relationships among systems, events, and variables.

5. Integrate thinking and doing to create environments and experiences that provide opportunities for people with ID-DD to learn from doing.

6. Integrate tacit (i.e., information grounded in people's values, norms, and expectations) and explicit (i.e., written reports, narratives, and databases) knowledge.

---

capital, community life context for quality of life, and managing for personal outcomes.

Social Capital

Recognizing the six emerging influences in scientific and social thinking summarized in Table 9.1 is an important step in reframing quality and rethinking quality improvement. However, using these new ideas requires a catalyst for action, and a practical approach to incorporating this new thinking into our work. We suggest that social capital, in theory and practice, offers one possibility for navigating the subtlety and ambiguity along our six continua:

Reductionism	Systems thinking
Mechanistic systems	Organic systems
Analysis	Synthesis
Planning	Self-organizing or emergence
Thinking	Engaging (doing)
Tacit knowledge	Explicit knowledge

Social capital refers to the connections among individuals: social networks and the norms of reciprocity and trust that arise from them (Adler & Kwan, 2002; Bolino, Turnley, & Bloodgood, 2002; Coleman, 1994; Putman, 2000; Putnam & Feldstein, 2003; Stone, 2003; Stone & Hughes, 2000, 2002; Tomer, 2003). These social networks have value. People in the networks trust one another and are inclined to do things for others in the social network (Bruhn, 2001; Seligman, 1997). The idea of reciprocity goes beyond returning a favor; the trust and reciprocity developed when someone has aided you generalizes to others in the social network, so that you may, in turn, help someone else in that network. Social capital works because of the transfer of benefits that flow from the trust, reciprocity, information, and cooperation growing out of the social network.

A worldwide body of literature indicates that social capital has a direct effect on social, economic, and individual development (Bradley & Kimmich, 2003; Gardner & Carran, 2005; Giles, Glonek, Luszcz, & Andrews, 2005; Putnam & Feldstein, 2003; Stone, 2003). This international literature on social capital has documented the beneficial outcomes of inclusion, community ties, reciprocity, and personal networks of trust. Consider that social capital (Putnam, 2000): (a) increases neighborhood stability; (b) helps to mitigate the insidious effects of socioeconomic disadvantage; (c) in the form of volunteering, entertaining, or regularly attending church or clubs, provides the happiness equivalent of getting a degree or more than doubling your income; (d) decreases the rates of illness and death; (e) rivals marriage and affluence as predictors of life happiness; and (f) reduces the instances of crime, teenage pregnancy, murder, child abuse, and welfare dependency.

The theory and practice of social capital appear when people form mutual support systems, personal futures planning sessions, circles of support, community ties, and social networks. Social capital serves as a catalyst in our thinking about quality and quality improvement in the field of ID-DD, because it brings together and emphasizes the following:

- *Systems thinking and synthesis.* Social capital is about networks and trusting relationships among networks and webs of people. A community of many trusting, knowledgeable, but isolated people is not rich in social capital.

- *Organic growth and emergence.* Social capital exists not in people but in the relationships between and among people. We can promote and encourage the development of social capital, but we cannot plan or control the nature of the resulting relationships. Networks and webs of interaction emerge.

- *Engaging others and learning through tacit and explicit knowledge exchange.* Social capital grows when people develop trusting and reciprocal relationships. Trust, mutual understanding, and shared values are often initially communicated through the exchange of tacit information. The converse corollary may also prove true, that social capital is a necessary condition for us to successfully transfer knowledge and human capital (Lesser, 2000). Only when people trust us can we pass on innovative ideas and transfer knowledge to them.

Social capital provides a catalyst because it is consistent with emerging scientific and social theory and practice. Social capital suggests how we can reconcile planning and emergence, mechanistic and organic systems of control, and systems of choice and self-determination with the need to promote health, safety, and human security. Our use of social capital as a construct does not apply to any conclusions about its rise and/or decline in general or to the many debates over its forms and types.

Federal, state, and community organizations cannot plan or create social capital. Instead, they can develop public policy, support communities, and help individuals find and nurture social networks based on trust and reciprocity. The role of the public sector, then, becomes one of planning, encouraging, and supporting the conditions that will spur the emergence of social capital networks and webs. The role of the support and service provider becomes one of connecting people with social capital networks in their own communities. Again, neither the public nor private sector can plan or control the emergence of social capital webs; they can only give people the opportunities and monitor progress.

The vocabulary of social capital offers a clear and generic alternative to the specialized language of disability services and programs. Researchers have documented the psychological, economic, social, medical, and educational benefits of social capital in all our lives, including those of people with ID-DD and their families, volunteers, service and support providers, and administrators. Increasing our social capital would benefit us all. With greater social capital, we will live healthier and happier, increase our community affiliations, and be able to exercise choice and self-determination.

Social capital offers a common meeting point for people receiving services and supports, families, employers, employees, and community organizations, both public and private.

With a clear focus on this concept, we can redefine the role and purpose of support and service programs to increase people's social capital. Organizations, both large and small, would be challenged to increase the social capital of people within the context of the community rather than the organization or program. In this way, people would have more allies and resources.

The concept of social capital also relates to employees. Organizations can enhance employee recruitment, retention, and development by building social capital. Recruitment, orientation, training, and retention would center on the potential employee's own social capital or the organization's capacity to develop social capital with the employee. The reality is that we can't expect our organizations to build social capital for people unless the employees experience productive social ties.

Social capital provides an additional management opportunity for leadership. We can manage our organizations by building social capital for all employees, increasing the richness of their ties to each other, their families, and the community. We can evaluate our organizational effectiveness by the impact we have on the social capital of our employees, as well as that of people we support.

We can also build and demonstrate accountability within our communities when we develop increased trustworthiness and social ties with public and private organizations. Enhancing our organizational capabilities through business-to-business ties increases our credibility and reciprocity with key opinion makers and community leaders. Moreover, trustworthiness and social ties have an attraction for families. Assisting families to develop social capital within our organizations and communities increases their connections to resources, broadening their network to incorporate more generic supports.

The common unifying task for the organization, formal or informal, is to build social capital for the community of interests it serves—people with disabilities, families, volunteers, and employees. The concept of social capital simplifies the measurement of quality. After demonstrating that we can deliver the basics in terms of health, safety, and security, we can measure the social capital of the individual, groups of people, or the whole organization. Social capital as a catalyst and an organizing construct goes beyond normalization, integration, or inclusion because it applies to everyone. We can use the same generic measure for all.

This organizing principle will take our thinking beyond organizations and programs. It will require organizations, formal and informal, large and small, to be responsible for building networks and connections for all their constituents. And we can best build social capital in communities, not within organizations and programs. Walls and barriers between people with disabilities, families, volunteers, employees, and the community will disappear as less formal structures replace the traditional hierarchies, job descriptions, and program structures.

A Community Life Context for Quality of Life

A second organizing principle stresses that an enhanced quality of life for people with ID-DD must occur within a community life context. By community life we mean the richness of resources that promote personal quality of life. Community life includes formal and informal supports for people in the areas of health care, housing, education, employment, transportation, and social capital. This emphasis on social capital, community life, and personal quality of life reflects our belief that we can only define quality in the context of community. We cannot focus solely on support or provider organizations, the informal network of friends and supporters, or the larger state or federal government.

During the 1990s, the field of ID-DD dramatically altered its definition of both *person* and *place* as it developed new quality measures. For example, the Council on Quality and Leadership (CQL) redefined person-directed quality in terms of *Personal Outcome Measures* (1993, 1997, 2000a) based on generic, QOL standards that apply to all people and aggregations of people. The Human Services Research Institute (HSRI) Core Indicators Project emphasized the normative aspects of personal QOL perceptions of people with disabilities, families, and providers (HSRI, 2003). In a similar manner, the American Association on Mental Retardation emphasized the connection between people, community, and individualized supports, and personal outcomes (Luckasson et al., 2002; Thompson et al., 2004).

Now we propose to again redefine place-based quality, redirecting it from the organization to the community. This change emphasizes the following:

- People and organizations are connected to other people and other organizations.

- Person-based quality is grounded in community. All places are both connected to, and part of, larger and more global places.

- Organizations connect citizens and their communities.

- Organizations can optimize the person-focused quality within the realities and possibilities of community life.

- Community life (community connections, relationships, and resources) supports personal quality of life and personal outcomes.

Organizations optimize both the goals and interests of person-defined quality of life within the opportunities and constraints of place-based quality in communities, and person-directed quality of life within the realities of place-based community life. For example, organizations assist people to find work they like within the existing job market. Bridging organizations influence communities and alter place-based community life to emphasize the characteristics and contributions of people. They may, for instance, show how realigned job duties better serve the needs of both the person and the employer. "Bridging" optimizes personal quality of life within place-based community life. The community life focus

- redefines place-based quality in the context of the community rather than that of the organization;

- enhances the options and resources for individual outcomes, self-determination, and individual financial budgeting;

- emphasizes the bridging role of organizations; organizations no longer serve the community by managing, controlling, or coordinating placements, contracts, or slots; and

- optimizes person-based quality of life within place-based community life.

The organization must also strive to optimize person and place-based quality for employees of organizations, community volunteers, and families of people with ID-DD. These people, most particularly direct-support professionals, play an important role in facilitating personal outcomes. The very same QOL indicators for people with ID-DD have great importance for people who support them, both paid and unpaid. To define these indicators, citizens ask, "What would make this community a healthier place?" The answer covers a wide range of community life indicators, such as transportation, jobs, housing, health care, education, and training. These community life factors also influence personal outcome planning and attainment, because they affect the availability and quality of the supports that facilitate personal outcomes. Organizations supplement their resources with those available through other community sources. They thus enhance outcomes for people by increasing community support capacity.

Community life is important because social support and the local environment and infrastructure influence the quality of life for people with ID-DD. The availability of health care, a strong economy and employment base, good transportation and communication, and a crime-free neighborhood with social and community patterns of support, tolerance, and diversity contribute to one's quality of life. In fact, these community variables may be as important as direct service for promoting quality of life for people (Gardner & Carran, 2005). To successfully develop community supports that facilitate personal outcomes, an organization needs to understand its surrounding community. To begin that process, the symbols for people and organizations shown in Figure 9.2 illustrate the reframing of quality and quality improvement (CQL, 2005d, 2005e).

The process of reframing quality and rethinking quality improvement involves realizing that historically there has been a transformation of the relationship among the people, organizations, and the community. The transformation begins in the not-too-distant past when human service systems focused primarily on the organizations that housed people with disabilities (depicted as Step 1 in Figure 9.3). Safe, clean facilities were built and managed to care for people 24 hours a day, 7 days a week.

Over time, the focus shifted to the individuals who were cared for by these organizations (Step 2, Figure 9.3). Practitioners and policy makers wanted to know what kinds of internal processes were necessary to ensure that the needs and desires of the "clients, patients, cases, or residents" were met. What kind of quality improvements and enhancements would ensure the highest quality services? How could social service and health service personnel best help "their individuals"?

With the consideration of the "person-in-the-organization" framework came the beginning realization that health and human service providers exist within the context of the broader community (Step 3, Figure 9.3). Each community is uniquely impacted by legislation, economic well-being, and social conditions. Hence, the focus moves to people who receive services from organizations that operate within a broader community. Many service organizations now operate in this manner. In other cases,

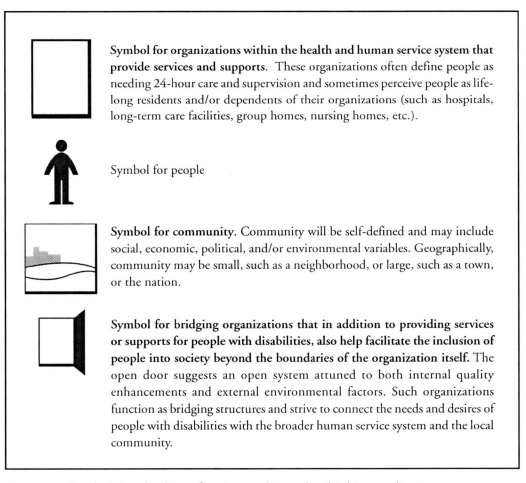

Figure 9.2. Symbols involved in reframing quality and rethinking quality improvement.

Note. Adapted from *Quality Measures 2005* and *Quality Measures 2005—Personal Outcome Measures* by the Council on Quality and Leadership, 2005, Towson, MD. Adapted with permission.

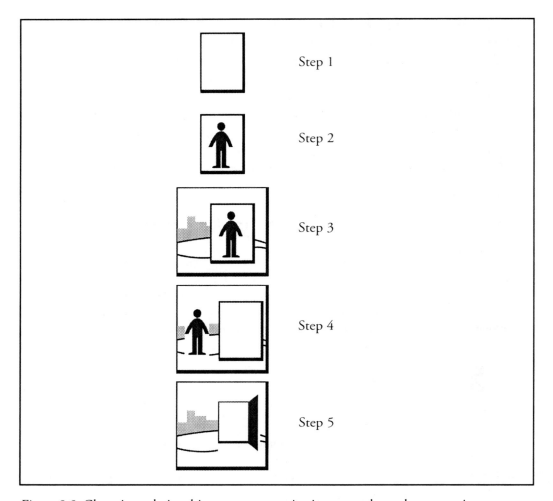

Figure 9.3. Changing relationships among organizations, people, and community.

Note. Adapted from *Quality Measures 2005* and *Quality Measures 2005—Personal Outcome Measures* by the Council on Quality and Leadership, 2005, Towson, MD. Adapted with permission.

however, as support personnel begin to see community context as integral to enhancing a person's quality of life, some individuals step out partially or fully from the confines and purview of organizations and live more inclusive and interdependent lives (Step 4). Thus they see the significance of facilitating and maximizing social capital and community supports. These organizations both enable individuals to realize their personal outcomes and respond to community factors that impact people with ID-DD (Step 5).

The processes depicted in Figures 9.2 and 9.3 reflect the changing relationships among people, communities, and organizations and suggest that many relationships can influence both personal outcomes and quality of community life. The relationships depicted in Figure 9.4 increase the importance of social capital and community life context for quality of life. As apparent as this transformation is, it occurs primarily in those organizations and systems that become bridges to the community; in the process they demonstrate our third organizing principle: managing for personal outcomes.

Managing for Personal Outcomes

Our third organizing principle is that continuous quality improvement requires a foundation in the values and principles derived from the QOL concept and a focus on obtaining QOL-related personal outcomes for people with ID-DD. But values by themselves are not significant to bring about those personal outcomes. In addition to the social capital and community context just described, organizations and systems need leadership and management strategies built on the critical success factors involved in making a personal outcome system work. As discussed in chapter 4 (see Figure 4.1) these factors are as follows:

- Strategy: a plan or method based on values and vision

- Execution: the performance of the plan or method

- Culture: the bond that unites and energizes people in execution

- Structure: roles, relationships, reporting, and feedback mechanisms that support culture

- Leadership: initiative and energy exercised by people, individually and collectively, through the structure

If organizations and systems are to manage for personal outcomes and thereby reduce the discrepancy between a person's desired outcomes and objective conditions within their community, managers must view their organization as a *bridge to the community*. As a bridge, an organization represents a means to the end for community inclusion, rather than an end in itself as a continuing provider of services and supports. Thus organizations as bridges:

- Define transitional and changing roles for themselves. Their roles and responsibilities become as varied as the people and the communities they link.

- Play a continuous role in connecting people to the community through individualized support plans that maximize social capital and natural supports.

- Display organic characteristics as they balance the dynamics of self-directed services with the evolving quality of community life. These decentralized structures and feedback are based on values, norms, and traditions rather than rules alone.

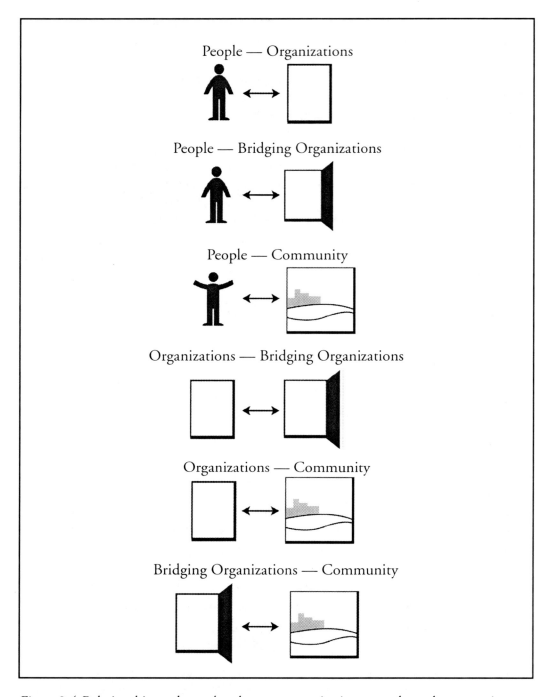

Figure 9.4. Relationships to be explored among organizations, people, and community.

Note. Adapted from *Quality Measures 2005* and *Quality Measures 2005—Personal Outcome Measures* by the Council on Quality and Leadership, 2005, Towson, MD. Adapted with permission.

Managing for QOL-related personal outcomes and transitioning to a bridging organization will require changes in leadership. As discussed in chapter 4, several leadership themes are particularly relevant in facilitating enhanced personal outcomes for people with ID-DD. Key aspects of these themes are summarized in Table 9.2.

TABLE 9.2
Key Leadership Themes That Facilitate Personal Outcomes

Servant leadership: Organizational leaders support staff members and other stakeholders in their efforts to facilitate and enhance personal outcomes.

Participant action research:

(a) Leaders from throughout the organization are participants in a continuous examination of quality of life.

(b) Leaders support action research that stresses the importance of taking action and then learning from those actions.

Community leadership: Organizational leaders recognize that lives and quality of life flourish in community and that organizations, by themselves, simply cannot offer the range of opportunities and life experiences available in the community and inherent in most QOL-related personal outcomes.

Cultural directors: Organizational leaders set and reinforce values, symbols, and priorities and pay conscious attention to those aspects of organizational life that maximize quality of life outcomes for people.

Invest in direct-support professional leadership: Direct-support professionals are directly responsible for delivering on the promises of basic assurances and personal outcomes. They are in the best position to: (a) connect and bridge to the community, and (b) facilitate those personal outcomes that require understanding of the person and a commitment to personal outcomes.

Summary

In summary, this chapter has stressed that if the quality of life of people with ID-DD is to be enhanced, organizations and systems need to move beyond traditional terms and concepts and focus on the true implications of the QOL concept. These implications force us to move beyond the person to the organization, system, and community. Basic to that transition is the need to reframe quality and rethink quality improvement.

Reframing quality involves more than understanding the conceptualization, measurement, and application of the QOL construct. In addition, it requires changing our mental models to reflect major changes in social policy and organizational practices. As noted throughout the chapter, these changes relate to: (a) a transformed vision of what constitutes the life possibilities of people with ID-DD including an emphasis on self-determination, community inclusion, and equity; (b) an ecological conception of disability that focuses on the person and his or her community; (c) the use of the QOL concept as a basis for best practices; and (d) the use of QOL-related outcomes information for multiple purposes, including quality assurance and quality improvement.

Responding to these changes requires a mental model or mind-set based on systems theory, organic organizations, creative synthesis, self-organizing and emergent systems, integrating doing and thinking, and integrating tacit and implicit knowledge. Similarly, rethinking quality improvement requires a different mind-set than organization-based services and supports and traditional quality assurance. Rather, it requires organizations and systems to think beyond their "places" and pursue three organizing principles: social capital, a community life context, and managing for personal outcomes. These three organizing principles reflect well the emerging movement *of being both in and of the community*.

We recognize the potential challenges (as well as opportunities) posed by the need for organizations and systems to reframe quality and rethink quality improvement. Moving forward to meet and overcome these challenges is addressed in the text's final chapter.

CHAPTER 10

Emerging Challenges and Opportunities

Introduction and Overview

At this point the reader is familiar with how the quality of life (QOL) concept has evolved from a sensitizing notion to its current use as a (a) multidimensional construct with measurable properties, (b) conceptual framework for assessing personal outcomes, (c) management orientation that guides quality improvement, and (d) change agent that at its core makes us think differently about people with intellectual disabilities and developmental disabilities (ID-DD) and how we might bring about change at the individual, organizational, systems, and community levels to enhance QOL-related personal outcomes. How we conceptualize, measure, and apply the concept has also evolved. As discussed throughout the text, a number of principles regarding the QOL concept have emerged over the past three decades (Brown, Keith, & Schalock, 2004; Schalock, 2005; Schalock et al., 2002):

- In regard to its conceptualization, quality of life is multidimensional and influenced by personal and environmental factors and their interactions; has the same components for all people; has both subjective and objective components; and is enhanced by self-determination, resources, purpose in life, and a sense of belonging.

- Measurement in quality of life involves the degree to which people have life experiences that they value; reflects the domains that contribute to a full and interconnected life; considers the contexts of physical, social, and cultural environments that are important to people; and includes measures of experiences both common to all humans and those unique to individuals.

- QOL application enhances well-being within cultural contexts and should be data-based; in addition, QOL principles should be the basis for interventions and support, and have a prominent place in professional education and training.

During the past three decades, we have seen analogous evolutionary patterns in those major concepts and areas we have discussed. Chief among these evolutionary changes has been the movement from:

- easy-to-identify-and-describe systems of public support for people with ID-DD to highly complex networks composed of widely varying levels and types of providers, settings, and structures;

- traditional standards and methods associated with compliance and documentation to a quality assessment and improvement methodology grounded in personal assurances and individual-referenced principles regarding the conceptualization, measurement, and application of the QOL concept;

- organization-based programs to community-based, individualized support systems;

- organizations as primary service providers to organizations as bridges to the community;

- mental models that stress reductionism, mechanistic systems, analysis, planning, thinking. and explicit knowledge to mental models that focus on systems thinking, organic and decentralized decision making, synthesis, self-organizing, doing, and a combination of tacit and explicit knowledge;

- management and leadership strategies that are organization or system oriented to strategies that involve managing for results, participant action research, community leadership, and cultural directors;

- external evaluation to making assessment and evaluation an ongoing, internal part of an organization's life;

- quality improvement as a management tool to quality improvement as an organization's or system's capacity to improve performance, person-referenced quality outcomes, and accountability through systematically collecting and analyzing data and information and implementing action strategies based on the analysis;

- quality assurance as a compliance or meeting-standards process to quality assurance as oversight that addresses a support's or provider's demonstrated ability to guarantee basic assurances in the areas of health, safety, and continuity.

These nine evolutionary changes require new ways of thinking and doing as we have addressed in the preceding nine chapters. They also present a number of challenges and opportunities to individuals, organizations, systems, and communities. The purpose of this concluding chapter is to discuss six of these important challenges and opportunities. Any insight we provide is based on our 110 years of collectively working in the field of ID-DD as well as our familiarity with the currently published literature and best practices. These six are (a) the QOL concept as a change agent, (b) QOL assessment and feedback as an integral part of how organizations and systems operate,

(c) consumers as key players, (d) organizations redefining their roles, (e) new management strategies, and (f) quality improvement as a continuous process.

The QOL Concept as a Change Agent

The QOL concept not only makes us think differently about people with ID-DD; it also makes us consider how we can use its conceptualization, measurement, and application principles to bring about change at the organizational and systems levels. In that regard, the use of QOL data or information for quality improvement requires an understanding that a person's quality of life as defined by personal outcomes and compared to community indicators is the lens through which one views, assesses, and understands the person's individual circumstances, and the performance of the organization and system. Thus using QOL as a change agent requires that we focus our efforts:

- At the individual level, on determining personal outcomes as defined by the person. Although we cannot have norms on how people define outcomes, we can measure whether they achieve those personal outcomes.

- At the organizational or systems level, on determining the predictors of aggregate personal outcomes. These identified predictors can then be used for quality improvement by engaging in "right-to-left thinking" that involves asking what needs to be in place within the organization and system for those personal outcomes to occur.

- At the community level, on establishing individualized systems of supports that maximize social capital, community life, and the attainment of personal outcomes.

These three mechanisms pose both challenges and opportunities for service or support providers and policy makers. The first is that QOL data or information remain sufficiently plastic and flexible that it can be translated into less constrained, more idiosyncratic situations and circumstances. The threat is that the QOL concept will become standardized and mechanistic and less individualized. Thus we need to maintain a dynamic balance between individuality and making it so prescriptive that is suffocates.

Second, it is important not to support the belief (and practice by some) that one gets to quality by more measurement. Measurement alone will not get us to where we want to get in regard to personal outcomes. We need to make change based on what we described in chapter 9 as "reframing quality" and "rethinking quality improvement" *and* good measurement and practices. As Boyle (2001) reminds us: "You cannot make sheep fatter by weighing them more often" (p. 10). QOL domains and indicators play a key role because they are based on a validated QOL model, and they determine the framework and general parameters for QOL measurement. Our challenge is to continue to question and validate through empirical research our assumptions, models, and their respective QOL-related indicators. A related need is to measure *only* what is really necessary, to prevent "respondent burnout."

The third challenge and opportunity is to determine whether the QOL concept as a service or supports delivery model applies equally well to other populations and systems. With the current emphasis on decategorization and generic services and supports, service providers and policy makers are searching for a generalizable model that will demonstrate measurability, reportability, and accountability. Data thus far suggest that the QOL concept, as summarized in the text, applies to other populations including seniors, individuals with mental or behavioral impairments, and students within special education (Gardner & Carran, 2005; National Core Indicators, 2005; Schalock & Verdugo, 2002).

QOL Assessment and Feedback as an Integral Part of Organizational and Systems Operations

QOL assessment is more than instruments and psychometrics. It is a process that begins with the individual as the key informant and ends with quality improvement. Thus one needs to think and *act beyond external monitoring and evaluation* (the historical approach) and *focus instead on an internal information collection and use process* that provides the basis for organizational development and quality improvement. As discussed in chapter 3 (see Table 3.2) a number of principles should guide this process, chiefly the following:

• Surveys should reflect what individuals value. Thus the person with ID-DD needs to be present from the beginning.

• Interviewers need to be competent, with competency demonstrated in a variety of ways. In this regard, it should not be overlooked that across a number of studies (e.g., Bonham et al., 2004; Schalock, Bonham, & Marchand, 2000; Schalock & Bonham, 2003) people with ID-DD have been trained to be competent QOL interviewers.

• The provider assumes responsibility for collecting the data. These data typically involve multiple data sources (e.g., personal outcomes, objective life conditions and circumstances, and proxy input) and other indicators (e.g., health, welfare, and rights) and linking that information to continuous program improvement.

• Collecting data and implementing quality-improvement strategies are viewed as a partnership among key stakeholders.

These four principles pose at least four challenges and opportunities. First, the development and use of an internal, individually referenced monitoring process in addition to an external monitoring process involves risks; getting "onboard" will take time for many organizations. In the meantime, external validation and the use of quality and performance indicators will be necessary—combined with technical assistance provided to organizations and systems around the following issues: (a) how to ask the right questions, (b) how to align the questions asked to data collection and analysis, (c) how to integrate the results, (d) how to act on the results, and (e) how to report quality improvement results.

Second, providers and policy makers need to see the relevance of using QOL assessment and feedback as an integral part of how their organization or system operates. In large part, this is the function of organizational or systems-level leadership in supporting other people in their efforts to facilitate personal outcomes for people with ID-DD.

Third, the costs (in terms of time, resources, and expertise) of collecting and analyzing multiple data sources need to be minimized by asking the right questions, making data-based decisions, and using integrated, computerized, real-time management information systems. Through these processes, organizations will be protected from being data rich but information poor.

The fourth challenge and opportunity involves research and evaluation activities. They need to involve all stakeholders and integrate the insight of consumers and providers with the technical expertise of the researcher or evaluator. Such collective efforts will be necessary to determine the significant predictors of personal outcomes and evaluate the overall effectiveness of the organization's or system's improvement on the attainment of personal outcomes.

Consumers as Key Players

Over the past three decades, we have experienced a transformed vision of what constitutes the life possibilities of individuals with ID-DD and the roles they should play in organizations and society. This transformed vision emphasizes self-determination, community inclusion, equity, and human potential. Throughout the text we have stressed that consumers identify their own personal outcomes, and that they need to be key players in organizational governance and participant action research.

There are at least three challenges and opportunities of consumers being key players. First, consumers need to have opportunities for being key players within organizations and systems. As discussed in chapters 4 and 7, the outcomes from these opportunities can be evaluated by affirmative answers to all the following questions: (a) Do people with ID-DD have the resources and supports to make their arguments and support their positions in debates and decision making? (b) In resolving conflict and reaching consensus within organizations and systems, do the interests of people with ID-DD match those of other stakeholders? (c) Do people with ID-DD hold the political power to set or influence the organization's or system's goals and mission? and (d) Are positive values, images, and symbols regarding people with ID-DD conveyed within the organization, system, and the community?

Second, collectively we need to reintegrate thinking and doing for people with ID-DD by involving them in action research. Two aspects of action research are key: (a) that learning is facilitated by doing, and (b) that consumers can play key roles in the planning, implementation or data collection, analysis, and application of research and evaluation efforts.

The third challenge and opportunity is to balance the impact of proxies, recognizing their strengths and limitations. As shown in Figure 3.1, their strengths lie in assessing objective QOL indicators, determining what supports are necessary and whether supports are present, and evaluating whether supports are working. They are least effective in assessing subjective QOL indicators and defining personal outcomes.

Organizations Redefining Their Roles

Organizations and systems providing services and supports to people with ID-DD are in the process of redefining their roles as they respond to the challenges of the quality revolution, the community-based movement, and the reform movement. As discussed throughout the text, these redefinitions are occurring along the following lines:

• Shifting from organization-based programs to community-based support systems

• Changing from organizations as primary service providers to organizations as bridges to the community

• Emphasizing the critical role that direct support professionals play in enhancing personal outcomes

These redefinitions are occurring within the context of two important phenomena: (a) the continued emergence of highly complex networks composed of widely varying levels and types of providers, settings, and structures, and (b) the increasing need to demonstrate measurability, reportability, and accountability. These phenomena and contextual issues pose three significant challenges and opportunities to organizations as they redefine their roles.

First, organizations will need to provide individualized supports to maximize personal outcomes within the context of community environments and community indicators. Providing these individualized supports requires at least a four-phase process: (a) developing a futures plan based on the individual's identified personal outcomes, (b) assessing the individual's profile and intensity of support needs, (c) developing an individual service plan, and (d) monitoring and evaluating as to whether the supports are present and effective in enhancing personal outcomes (Luckasson et al., 2002; Thompson et al., 2004). The effectiveness of this process needs to be evaluated in reference to both the individual's standards and how the person's objective life conditions and circumstances compare to his or her community's indicators. This process will require organizations to develop the internal monitoring activities discussed earlier and to look more to the community for relevant standings and benchmarks.

The second challenge is to understand the community to which the organization is bridging. Nationally and internationally current policy and practices are designed to promote the acceptance, integration, and inclusion of people with ID-DD into their communities. This trend is based on the premise that people want and have a right to full community inclusion and membership. Its successful fulfillment requires not just the infrastructure (i.e., organizations as bridges to the community), but also a clear understanding of community attitudes about people with ID-DD and attitude change. In that regard, Myers, Ager, Kerr, and Myles (1998) have identified three classes of attitudes that influence how community members interact with and include or exclude people with ID-DD:

- A preparedness to engage with people as consumers, neighbors, or friends. This attitude needs to be supported and reinforced.

- A lack of awareness about individuals with ID-DD. This attitude needs to be addressed by providing information about the positiveness and potential of these individuals.

- A wariness or even hostility regarding the idea of community integration. This attitude can best be changed by identifying individuals in the community who can be agents of positive change. As Reinders (1999) suggests, "without the influence of people who have sufficient moral character to care, rights can do little to sustain the mentally disabled and their families" (p. 23).

The third challenge and opportunity relates to the role played by the direct-support professional. As organizations become more horizontal and engage in right-to-left thinking as part of their quality improvement process, direct support professionals will play an increasingly valued role in the planning, delivery, and evaluation of services and supports. In this regard, two things should be remembered: First, social capital applies not only to people with ID-DD, but also to employees and their families. Second, managers need to recognize the tacit knowledge that direct-support professionals have in quality improvement and enhancing personal outcomes. The caveat is that they understand the concept of quality of life and its conceptualization (in regard to core domains and indicators), measurement (in regard to personal outcomes), and application (in regard to reducing the discrepancy between defined personal outcomes and community indicators). This increased understanding should be a priority in human resource development activities.

As organizations redefine their roles, it is important for them to understand the characteristics of successful organization and systems-level change. Chief among these characteristics (Schalock, 2001; Schalock & Bonham, 2003) are the following:

- Organizational level: openness to risk, shared values that drive services, ongoing process of self-evaluation, linkage to external resources, holistic focus on consumer needs, direct-staff roles in organizational goals and decision making, and an emphasis on quality improvement

- Systems-level: flexibility and innovation, incentives to agencies to expand community living and community options, community support and advocacy, systems-level goals and data collection, and using that information for continuous systems-level quality improvement

New Management Strategies

Chapter 6 described how the service delivery system is becoming more diffuse, less centralized, and more individualized. The net result of this change is that there is more ambiguity and less certainty. Thus, as discussed in chapters 4 and 9, old-line chains of command and mechanistic management models don't work any longer. Currently we are also seeing:

- management and leadership strategies that involve managing for results, participant action research, community leadership, and cultural directors;

- mental models that focus on systems thinking, organic and decentralized decision making, synthesis, self-organizing, doing (rather then merely thinking and planning), and combining tacit and explicit knowledge;

- data-based decision making in which data and information are systematically collected and analyzed by the organization, and action strategies are developed based on the analysis.

These three developments contain at least three challenges and opportunities. First, managers need to employ strategies that reflect current realities. In Table 9.1 we suggested six such strategies characterizing a "reframing quality" and "rethinking quality improvement" mental model: (a) embrace systems theory; (b) employ an organic approach that emphasizes decentralized decision-making responsibility, increases the autonomy and power of people using services, and decreases the role and power of professionals and bureaucrats; (c) focus on a synthetic process that brings together individual components to better understand the larger phenomenon; (d) develop self-organizing systems that emphasize network and web relationships among systems, events, and variables; (e) integrate thinking and doing; and (f) integrate tacit and explicit knowledge.

Second, managers need to move from "information age" to "conceptual age" in their thinking. In the recent book *A Whole New Mind: Moving From the Information to Conceptual Age*, Daniel Pink (2005) identifies six management aptitudes needed in the 21st century:

- Design: The product must be more than functional; it must also be beautiful, whimsical, or emotionally engaging.

- Story: A compelling narrative is essential for persuasion.
- Symphony: The ability to piece together into a winning combination; what's in greatest demand today isn't analysis, but synthesis.
- Empathy: The need to move beyond logic and to understand what makes people forge relationships and care for others.
- Play: The need to work *and* play.
- Meaning: People need to be free to pursue purpose, transcendence, and fulfillment.

The third challenge and opportunity relates to the position in which many managers find themselves: caught between consumers, state and federal regulators, and the state licensing or regulatory process. Here managers of both organizations and systems need to realize that shifting to a data-based QOL model with its emphasis on assessment and feedback will take both time and a commitment to new management strategies. An important part of that process is to appreciate the reality of a learning curve that can be accelerated by understanding: (a) the QOL concept and its philosophical and empirical basis (see chaps. 1 & 2), (b) how to assess personal outcomes (see chaps. 3, 5, & 7), and (c) how to use multilevel subject and objective indicators for quality improvement (see chaps. 3, 4, 8, & 9).

We recognize that these three challenges and our suggestions in reference to each may well represent new ideas and ways of thinking and doing. We also appreciate the fact that the adoption of a new idea is complex. According to Rogers (1995), for example, the rate of adoption of a new idea is explained by five attributes of the innovation or new idea itself: (a) whether the innovation or idea is seen as an advantage over the previous idea; (b) whether it is consistent with the values, past experiences, and needs of potential adopters; (c) whether it is perceived as overly complex; (d) whether it is possible to do a small tryout of parts of the innovation; and (e) whether the results of the innovation can be observed.

Quality Improvement as a Continuous Process

We have also stressed repeatedly that quality improvement is not quality assurance.

- Quality assurance refers to quality oversight that addresses a support's or service provider's demonstrated ability to guarantee basic assurances in the areas of health, safety, and continuity. Thus quality assurance precedes quality improvement and focuses on remediation and basic assurances.
- Quality improvement refers to an organization's or system's capacity to improve performance and accountability through systematically collecting and analyzing data and information and implementing action strategies based on the analysis. Its

goal is to improve the quality of life of individuals through the enhancement of policies, practices, training, technical assistance, and other organizational and/or systems-level supports.

As shown in Figure 10.1, our approach to quality improvement is based on reducing the discrepancy between assessed personal outcomes and community indicators. The systematic assessment of personal outcomes and their comparison with community, QOL-related indicators provide the data and information for analysis and subsequent use in the quality-improvement process. This approach to quality improvement is consistent with the shift from traditional standards and methods associated with compliance and documentation to a quality assessment and improvement methodology grounded in personal assurances and individual-referenced QOL conceptualization, measurement, and application principles. It also involves all major stakeholders as suggested here:

• Individuals articulate the way in which outcomes are achieved by defining for themselves relevant personal outcomes.

• Organizations respond to the quality-improvement imperative by reducing the discrepancy noted in Figure 10.1 through systematically collecting and analyzing data and information and implementing action strategies such as opportunity development, maximizing social capital, or providing individualized supports.

• Systems support organizational efforts or action strategies and provide the legal and regulatory structures to ensure their successful implementation.

Approaching quality improvement as a continuous process of reducing the

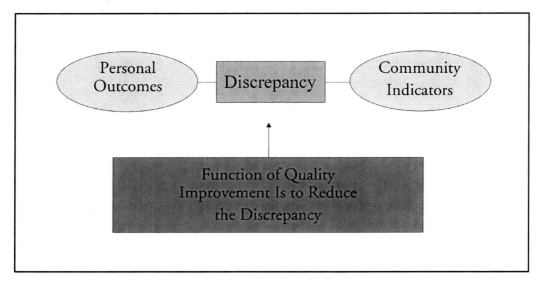

Figure 10.1. Quality-improvement process.

discrepancy between assessed personal outcomes and community indicators presents organizations and systems with at least four challenges and opportunities. First, they need to integrate personal and aggregate outcome indicators into a seamless, data information system. As discussed in parts 2 and 3, personal outcomes that define quality of life in regard to core domains and indicators can be (a) aggregated at the provider and/or systems level, and (b) complemented by other systems-level indicators (e.g., staff turnover, health indicators). To prevent information overload and provide meaningful analysis, synthesis, and use, selected indicators should meet those 10 criteria listed in Table 2.8 and described further in chapter 7. Quality indicators should (a) have face validity; (b) be measurable and psychometrically sound; (c) be conceptually related to a validated QOL model; (d) have potential for improvement; (e) be those the provider has some control over; and (f) be comprehensive.

Second, an organization's quality-improvement process needs to be accountable and based on data or information that is reliable, valid, and based on people's priorities. One model for doing this has been the quality framework prepared by the Centers for Medicare and Medicaid Services (see Figure 6.2) that includes three critical functions:

- Discovery: engaging in procedures to collect data and information about participant experiences, to access the ongoing implementation of the program, identify strengths, and provide other opportunities for improvement

- Remediation: taking action to remedy specific problems or concerns that arise

- Quality improvement: using data and quality information to engage in actions that result in improved program operatives

Third, all stakeholders need to think differently about the purpose and use of comparisons. Here we offer the following three suggestions: (a) individually defined personal outcomes cannot be compared (in terms of good or bad, relevant or irrelevant) to others, even though they can be aggregated at the organizational or systems level and used for reporting and statistical analyses such as determining outcome predictors; (b) at the systems level, risk adjustment (see chap. 7) is required for comparability across different jurisdictions, whereas benchmarks regarding aggregate personal outcomes can be used for quality improvement; and (c) at the systems level, one should not compare an individual's definition of personal outcomes or one program's outcomes with another; rather, the emphasis should be on measuring the accomplishments of a set of personal outcomes from a system's perspective.

The fourth challenge and opportunity is to demonstrate the advantage of using quality improvement as a continuous process. Because this approach to quality improvement represents change, it is important to underscore our understanding that going forward means change and that change is not easy. Change does not occur in a vacuum, because it takes place within an already well defined and established context. Our challenge as authors and implementers is to understand and explain clearly to all stakeholders how quality improvement as a continuous process and one based on a data-based QOL model should in time allow organizational and systems managers to answer in the affirmative each of the following five questions posed by DeJager (2001): (a) Why is the old status no longer sufficient? (b) What will it cost (in resources, expertise, and time) to make the transition from the old to the new? (c) Is this "cost of transition" justified by the incremental focusing on quality outcomes and performance enhancement? (d) Does the proposed change support and reinforce core values? and (e) Are key stakeholders involved in the process?

Quality of Life for People With ID-DD: Going Forward

In the end, this book reflects a journey that begins with determining what is important to individuals with ID-DD and then developing the services, supports, and quality-improvement strategies that enhance personal outcomes within a community context. It's a journey that requires people to think differently about the QOL concept and its conceptualization, measurement, and application. Furthermore, it's a journey that involves challenges and opportunities related to (a) using the QOL concept as a change agent, (b) integrating QOL assessment and feedback as an integral part of organizational and systems operations, (c) supporting consumers to be key players within organizations and systems, (d) redefining organizations' roles, (e) exhibiting new management strategies, and (f) viewing quality improvement as a continuous process.

When we began writing this book, we felt strongly (as we still do) that the large-scale adoption of a person-centered approach to basic assurances and QOL assessment would require a data-based quality (of life) model around which organizations and systems could organize their services and supports and on which they could base their quality-improvement process. That model has emerged throughout the text as we have (a) indicated how the QOL concept has become a change agent; (b) synthesized current research and literature in the area of quality of life and its measurement and how the concept has influenced management strategies, organizational design, systems change, and leadership; (c) provided examples of how the QOL concept can be operationalized, measured, and applied at the individual, organizational, and systems level; (d) showed how QOL-related personal outcomes (singularly and aggregate) can be used to facilitate quality improvement and enhance personal outcomes; and (e) suggested ways that organizations and systems can move beyond traditional terms and concepts to a QOL focus with its emphasis on the achievement of personal outcomes within the community context.

Our hope is that we will continue to go forward in our respective journeys, overcoming the challenges and grasping the opportunities associated with applying the QOL concept across individuals, organizations, communities, and systems. If that is the case, our journey has been both productive and worthwhile.

References

Academy of Human Resource Development. (1999). *Standards on ethics and integrity.* Baton Rouge, LA: Author.

Accreditation Council on Services for People With Disabilities. (1993). *Outcome based performance measures: Procedures manual.* Towson, MD: Author.

Adler, P. S., & Kwan, S. W. (2002). Social capital: Prospects for a new concept. *Academy of Management Review, 27*(1), 17–40.

American Evaluation Association Task Force on Guiding Principles for Evaluation. (1995). Guiding principles for evaluators. In W. R. Shadish, D. L. Newman, M. A. Scheirer, & C. Wye (Eds.), *Guiding principles for evaluators* (New directions for program evaluation, Vol. 66; pp. 19–26). San Francisco: Jossey-Bass.

Americans With Disabilities Act of 1990, 42 U.S.C.A. § 12101 *et seq.* (West 1993).

Anastasi, A., & Urbina, S. (1997). *Psychological testing* (7th ed.). Upper Saddle River, NJ: Prentice-Hall.

Andrews, A. B. (2004). Start at the end: Empowerment evaluation product planning. *Evaluation and Program Planning, 27*(3), 275–285.

Andrews, F. M., & Whithey, S. B. (1976). *Social indicators of well-being: Americans' perception of life quality.* New York: Plenum Press.

Antaki, C., & Rapley, M. (1996). Questions and answers to psychological assessment schedules: Hidden troubles in "quality of life" interviews. *Journal of Intellectual Disability Research, 40,* 421–437.

Ashbaugh, J., Banks, S., & Taub, S. (1999). *Outcome adjustment, project technical report: Core Indicators Project.* Cambridge, MA: Human Services Research Institute.

Baldrige National Quality Program. (2005). *Criteria for performance excellence.* Milwaukee, WI: American Society for Quality Control.

Bardach, E. (1977). *The implementation game: What happens after a bill becomes law.* Cambridge, MA: MIT Press.

Baron, S., Field, J., & Schuller, T. (Eds.). (2000). *Social capital: Critical perspectives.* Oxford: Oxford University Press.

Beauchamp, T. L., & Childress, J. F. (1983). *Principles of biomedical ethics* (2nd ed.). New York: Oxford University Press.

Bolino, M. C., Turnley, W. H., & Bloodgood, J. M. (2002). Citizenship behavior and the creating of social capital in organizations. *Academy of Management Review, 27*(4), 505–522.

Bolman, L., & Deal, T. (2003). *Reframing organizations: Artistry, choice and leadership* (3rd ed.). San Francisco: Jossey-Bass.

Bonham, S. G., Basehart, S., & Marchand, C. B. (2003). *Ask Me! FY 2003 report: The quality of life of Marylanders with developmental disabilities receiving DDA funded support.* Baltimore: The ARC of Maryland.

Bonham, S. G., Basehart, S., Schalock, R. L., Marchand, C. B., Kirchner, N., & Rumenap, J. M. (2004). Consumer-based quality of life assessment: The Maryland Ask Me! Project. *Mental Retardation, 42*(5), 338–355.

Bossidy, L., Charan, R., & Burck, C. (2002). *Execution: The discipline of getting things done.* New York: Crown.

Boyle, D. (2001). *The sum of our discontent: Why numbers make us irrational.* New York: Texere.

Bradley, V. J., & Kimmich, M. (2003). *Quality enhancement in developmental disabilities.* Baltimore: Paul H. Brookes.

Brown, I., Keith, K. D., & Schalock, R. L. (2004). Quality of life conceptualization, measurement, and application: Validation of the SIRG-QOL consensus principles. *Journal of Intellectual Disability Research, 48*(4–5), 451.

Bruhn, J. G. (2001). *Trust and the health of organizations.* New York: Plenum.

Bruininks, R. H., Hill, B. K., Weatherman, R. F., & Woodcock, R. W. (1986). *Inventory for client and agency planning.* Itasca, IL: Riverside.

Burns, T., & Stalker, G. M. (1961). *The management innovation.* London: Tavistok.

Bushe, G. (1998). Appreciate inquiry with teams. *Organization Development Journal, 16*(3), 41–50.

Campbell, A., Converse, P. E., & Rogers, W. L. (1976). *The quality of American life: Perceptions, evaluations, and satisfaction.* New York: Russell Sage.

Capra, F. (1982). *The turning point: Science, society, and the rising culture.* New York: Bantam.

Capra, F. (1991). *The Tao of physics: An exploration of the parallels between modern physics and Eastern mysticism.* Boston: Shambhala.

Capra, F. (1996). *The web of life: A new scientific understanding of living systems.* New York: Doubleday, Anchor.

Capra, F. (2002). *The hidden connections: Integrating the biological, cognitive and social dimensions of life into a science of sustainability.* New York: Doubleday.

Chambers, R. (1997). *Whose reality counts? Putting the first last.* London: ITDS.

Chelimsky, E., & Shadish, W. R. (1995). *Evaluation for the 21st century: A handbook.* Thousand Oaks, CA: Sage.

Chen, H. T. (1990). *Theory-driven evaluations.* Newbury Park, CA: Sage.

Christianson, L. (2004). *Using NCI to measure performance at the Regional Center of Orange County.* PowerPoint presentation at the National Reinventing Quality Conference, Philadelphia.

Coleman, J. S. (1990). *Foundations of social theory.* Cambridge, MA: Harvard University Press.

Coleman, J. S. (1994). *Foundations of social theory.* Cambridge, MA: Belknap Press.

Converse, J. M., & Presser, S. (1986). *Survey questions: Handcrafting the standardized questionnaire.* New Delhi, India: Sage.

Cooperrider, D. L., & Srivastva, S. (1987). Appreciative inquiry into organizational life. *Research in Organizational Change and Development, 5,* 129–169.

Council on Quality and Leadership. (1993). *Outcome based performance measures.* Towson, MD: Author.

Council on Quality and Leadership. (1997). *Personal outcome measures.* Towson, MD: Author.

Council on Quality and Leadership. (2000a). *Accreditation: A quality review and enhancement process.* Towson, MD: Author.

Council on Quality and Leadership. (2000b). *Assessment workbook for use with the personal outcome measures: 2000 edition.* Towson, MD: Author.

Council on Quality and Leadership. (2000c). *Importance Satisfaction Map™.* Towson, MD: Author.

Council on Quality and Leadership. (2000d). *Personal outcome measures: 2000 edition.* Towson, MD: Author.

Council on Quality and Leadership. (2000e). *Personal outcome measures for children and youth.* Towson, MD: Author.

Council on Quality and Leadership. (2000f). *Personal outcome measures in consumer-directed behavioral health.* Towson, MD: Author.

Council on Quality and Leadership. (2000g). *Personal outcome measures for families with young children.* Towson, MD: Author.

Council on Quality and Leadership. (2001). *Life support: Connecting choices—an action workbook for consumers of behavioral health services.* Towson, MD: Author.

Council on Quality and Leadership. (2002). *Life support: Connecting choices—an action workbook—my choices, my goals, my chance.* Towson, MD: Author.

Council on Quality and Leadership. (2005a). *Basic assurances.* Towson, MD: Author.

Council on Quality and Leadership. (2005b). *Personal outcome measures.* Towson, MD: Author.

Council on Quality and Leadership. (2005c). *Social capital index.* Towson, MD: Author.

Council on Quality and Leadership. (2005d). *Quality measures 2005.* Towson, MD: Author.

Council on Quality and Leadership. (2005e). *Quality measures 2005—Personal outcome measures.* Towson, MD: Author.

Council on Quality and Leadership. (2005f). *National database.* Accessible online at: www.cql.org

Cronbach, L. J. (1951). Coefficient alpha and the internal structure of tests. *Psychometrika, 16*(3), 297–334.

Cummins, R. A. (1997a). Assessing quality of life. In R. I. Brown (Ed.), *Assessing quality of life for people with disabilities: Models, research, and practice* (pp. 16–150). London: Stanley Thornes.

Cummins, R. A. (1997b). *Comprehensive QOL Scale Intellectual/Cognitive Disability manual* (5th ed.). Melbourne, Australia: Deakin University, School of Psychology.

Cummins, R. A. (1998). The second approximation to an international standard for life satisfaction. *Social Indicators Research, 43,* 307–334.

Cummins, R. A. (2003). *Personal Well-Being Index: Intellectual Disability.* Melbourne: Deakin University, Australian Centre on Quality of Life.

Cummins, R. A. (2004a). Instruments for assessing quality of life. In J. H. Hogg & A. Langa (Eds.), *Approaches to the assessment of adults with intellectual disabilities: A service provider's guide.* London: Blackwell.

Cummins, R. A. (2004b). Issues in the systematic assessment of quality of life. In J. H. Hogg & A. Langa (Eds.), *Approaches to the assessment of adults with intellectual disabilities: A service provider's guide.* London: Blackwell.

Cummins, R. A., & Lau, A. L. D. (2004). The motivation to maintain subjective well-being: A homeostatic model. *International Review of Research in Mental Retardation, 28,* 255–301.

Davenport, T. H., & Prusak, L. (1998). *Working knowledge: How organizations manage what they know.* Cambridge, MA: Harvard Business School Press.

Deal, T. E., & Kennedy, A. A. (1999). *The new corporate cultures: Revitalizing the workplace after downsizing, mergers, and reengineering.* Reading, MA: Perseus.

Deci, E. L. (2004). Promoting intrinsic motivation and self-determination in people with mental retardation. *International Review of Research in Mental Retardation, 28,* 1–29.

DeJager, P. (2001, May–June). Resistance to change: A new view of an old problem. *The Futurist*, 24–27.

Denzin, N. K., & Lincoln, Y. S. (Eds.). (2000). *Handbook of qualitative research* (2nd ed.). Thousand Oaks, CA: Sage.

Dewa, C. S., Horgan, S., Russell, M., & Keates, J. (2001). What? Another form? The process of measuring and comparing service utilization in a community mental health program model. *Evaluation and Program Planning, 24*, 239–247.

Donaldson, S. E., & Gooler, L. E. (2003). Theory-driven evaluation in action: Lessons from a $20 million statewide work and health initiative. *Evaluation and Program Planning, 26*(4), 355–366.

Emerson, E. (2005, April 26). In defense of objective social indicators. Paper presented at the Vancouver SIRG-QOL Roundtable, Vancouver, BC, Canada.

Feinstein, C., & Caruso, G. (2003). The Pennsylvania experience. In V. Bradley & M. Kimmich (Eds.), *Quality enhancement in developmental disabilities: Challenges and opportunities in a changing world* (pp. 175–190). Baltimore: Paul H. Brookes.

Felce, D. (1997). Defining and applying the concept of quality of life. *Journal of Intellectual Disability Research, 41*(2), 126–135.

Felce, D., & Perry, J. (1996). Assessment of quality of life. In R. L. Schalock (Ed.), *Quality of life. Vol. 1: Conceptualization and measurement* (pp. 63–73). Washington, DC: American Association on Mental Retardation.

Ferdinand, R., & Smith, M. A. (2002). *2002 Nebraska developmental disabilities provider profiles*. Lincoln: The ARC of Nebraska.

Finlay, W. M. L., & Lyons, E. (2002). Acquiescence in interviews with people who have mental retardation. *Mental Retardation, 40*(1), 14–29.

Fisher, R., & Ury, W. (1988). *Getting to yes: Negotiating agreement without giving in.* New York: Penguin.

Fishman, D. B. (2003). Postmodernism comes to program evaluation IV: A review of *Denzin and Lincoln's Handbook of Qualitative Research* (2nd ed.). *Evaluation and Program Evaluation, 26*(4), 415–420.

Flannery, T. P., Hofrichter, D. A., & Platten, P. E. (1996). *People, performance and pay.* New York: Free Press.

Fox, M. H., Kim, K., & Ehrenkrantz, D. (2002). Developing comprehensive statewide disability information systems. *Journal of Disability Policy Studies, 13*(3), 171–179.

French, W., & Bell, C. H. (1998). *Organization development. Behavioral science interventions for organization improvement* (6th ed.). New York: Prentice-Hall.

Friedman, V. (2001). Action science: Creating communities of inquiry in communities of practice. In P. Reason & H. Bradbury (Eds.), *Handbook of action research: Participative inquiry and practice* (pp. 159–171). Thousand Oaks, CA: Sage.

Gallivan, J. (2005). State of Maine: Quality management and National Core Indicators. PowerPoint presentation at the National Reinventing Conference, Philadelphia.

Gardner, J. F. (1995). Maintaining quality and managing change: Administration in transition. In O. C. Karan & S. Greenspan (Eds.), *Community rehabilitation services for people with disabilities.* Boston: Butterworth-Heinemann.

Gardner, J. F. (2002). The evolving social context for quality in services and supports. In R. L. Schalock, P. C. Baker, & M. D. Croser (Eds.), *Embarking on a new century: Mental retardation at the end of the 20th century* (pp. 67–80). Washington, DC: American Association on Mental Retardation.

Gardner, J. F. (2003). *Challenging tradition: Measuring quality through personal outcomes.* Towson, MD: The Council on Quality and Leadership.

Gardner, J. F., & Carran, D. (2005). Attainment of personal outcomes by people with developmental disabilities. *Mental Retardation, 43*(3), 157–174.

Gardner, J. F., Carran, D. T., & Nudler, S. (2001). Measuring quality of life and quality of services through personal outcome measures: Implications for public policy. *International Review of Research in Mental Retardation, 24*, 75–100.

Gardner, J. F., & Nudler, S. (1997). Beyond compliance to responsiveness: Accreditation reconsidered. In R. L. Schalock (Ed.), *Quality of life. Vol. 2: Application to persons with disabilities* (pp. 135–148). Washington, DC: American Association on Mental Retardation.

Gardner, J. F., & Nudler, S. (Eds.). (1999). *Quality performance in human services: Leadership, vision, and values.* Baltimore: Paul H. Brookes.

Gardner, J. F., Nudler, S., & Chapman, M. (1997). Personal outcome measures of quality. *Mental Retardation, 35*, 295–305.

Gettings, R. M., & Bradley, V. J. (1997). *Core indicators project.* Alexandria, VA: National Association of State Directors of Developmental Disabilities Services.

Giles, L. C., Glonek, G. F. V., Luszcz, M. A., & Andrews, G. R. (2005). Effects of social networks on 10-year survival in very old Australians: The Australian longitudinal study of aging. *Journal of Epidemiology and Community Health. 59*, 574–579.

Government Performance and Results Act of 1993 (GPRA). Washington, DC: Government Printing Office.

Greenleaf, R. K. (1991). *Servant leadership.* Mahwah, NJ: Paulist.

Hakes, J. E. (2001). Can measuring results produce results: One manager's view. *Evaluation and Program Planning, 24*, 319–327.

Harner, C. J., & Heal, L. (1993). Multifactorial Lifestyle Satisfaction Scale (MLSS): Psychometric properties of an interview schedule for assessing personal satisfaction of adults with limited intelligence. *Research in Developmental Disabilities, 14*, 221–236.

Hayden, M. F., & Nelis, T. (2002). Self-advocacy. In R. L. Schalock, P. C. Baker, & M. D. Croser (Eds.), *Embarking on a new century: Mental retardation at the end of the 20th century* (pp. 221–234). Washington, DC: American Association on Mental Retardation.

Heal, L. W. & Sigelman, C. K. (1996). Methodological issues in quality of life measurement. In R. L. Schalock (Ed.), *Quality of Life. Vol. 1: Conceptualization and measurement* (pp. 91–104). Washington, DC: American Association on Mental Retardation.

Helgesen, S. (1995). *The web on inclusion.* New York: Doubleday, Currency.

Hemp, R., & Braddock, D. (1990). Accreditation of Developmental Disabilities Programs. In V. Bradley & H. Bersani (Eds.), *Quality assurances for individuals with developmental disabilities: It's everybody's business* (pp. 150–172). Baltimore: Paul H. Brookes.

Herr, S. S., O'Sullivan, J., & Hogan, C. (2002). A friend in court: The Association's role and judicial trends. In R. L. Schalock, P. C. Baker, & M. D. Croser (Eds.), *Embarking on a new century: Mental retardation at the end of the 20th century* (pp. 27–44). Washington, DC: American Association on Mental Retardation.

Hodges, S. P., & Hernandez, M. (1999). How organizational culture influences outcome information utilization. *Evaluation and Program Planning, 22*, 183–197.

House, E. R. (1991). Research in realism. *Educational Researcher, 20*(6), 2–9.

Hughes, C., Hwang, B., Kim, J., Eiseman, L. T., & Killian, D. J. (1995). Quality of life in applied research: A review and analysis of empirical measures. *American Journal on Mental Retardation, 99*, 623–641.

Human Services Research Institute. (2003). *National core indicators: A growing commitment.* Cambridge, MA: Author.

Human Services Research Institute. (2004). *Consumer outcomes: Phase VI final report.* Retrieved October 28, 2004, from http://www.hsri.org/docs/786_P6_consumer2004_final pdf

Human Services Research Institute & National Association of State Directors of Developmental Disabilities Services. (2003). *National core indicators: 5 years of performance measurement.* Cambridge, MA, & Alexandria, VA: Authors.

Individuals With Disabilities Act of 1990 (IDEA), Pub. L. No. 101-476.

Institute for Community Inclusion. (2005). *StateData.info.* Retrieved June 2, 2005, from http://www.statedata.info

International Organization for Standardization. (2003). *ISO 9000 quality management: ISO standards compendium.* New York: American National Standards Institute.

Isenberg, D. (1984, November–December). How senior managers think. *Harvard Business Review,* pp. 81–90.

Jaskulski, T. (1991). *Affecting the quality of services: Perspectives on quality and home and community based services for people with developmental disabilities.* Columbia, MD: Jaskulski & Associates.

Jenaro, C., Verdugo, M. A., Caballo, C., Balboni, G., Lachapelle, Y., Otrebski, W., & Schalock, R. L. (2005). Cross-cultural study of person-centered quality of life domains and indicators: A replication. *Journal of Intellectual Disability Research, 49*(10), 734–739.

Johnson, R. B. (1998). Toward a theoretical model of evaluation utilization. *Evaluation and Program Planning, 21,* 93–110.

Joyce, W., Nohria, N., & Roberson, B. (2003). *What really works: The 4 + 2 formula for sustained business success.* New York: Harper Business.

Kaplan, R. S. (1996). *The balanced scorecard: Translating strategy into action.* Cambridge, MA: Harvard Business School Press.

Kaplan, S. A., & Garrett, K. E. (2005). The use of logic models by community-based initiatives. *Evaluation and Program Planning, 28*(2), 167–172.

Karon, S. L., & Bernard, S. (2002). *Development of operational definitions of quality indicators for Medicaid Services to people with developmental disabilities.* Submitted to U.S. Department of Health & Human Services, Centers for Medicare & Medicaid Services, January 1, 2002.

Karon, S. L., Stegemann, A. D., & Barnard, S. (2003, October). *Technical summation report.* Submitted to Centers for Medicare and Medicaid Services. Triangle Park, NJ: RTI International.

Keith, K. D., & Bonham, G. S. (2005). The use of quality of life data at the organization and systems level. *Journal of Intellectual Disability Research, 49*(10), 799–805.

Kelly, K. (1995). *Out of control: The new biology of machines, social systems, and the economic world.* Reading, MA: Addison-Wesley.

Kotter, J. (1982). *The general managers.* New York: Free Press.

Krogh, K. (1995). Developing a partnership agreement. In J. Pivik (Ed.), *Facilitating collaborative research between consumers and researchers* (pp. 69–75). Ottawa, ON, Canada: Institute for Rehabilitation Research and Development.

Kuhn, T. (1961). *The structure of scientific revolutions.* Chicago: University of Chicago Press.

Langer, E. J. (1997). *The power of mindful learning.* Reading, MA: Addison-Wesley.

Larson, S. A., Lakin, K. C., & Hewitt, A. S. (2002). Direct service professionals: 1975–2000. In R. L. Schalock, P. C. Baker, & M. D. Croser (Eds.), *Embarking on a new century: Mental retardation at the end of the 20th century* (pp. 203–220). Washington, DC: American Association on Mental Retardation.

Lesser, E. L. (Ed.). (2000). *Knowledge and social capital: Foundations and applications.* Boston: Butterworth Heinemann.

Luckasson, R., Borthwick-Duffy, S., Buntinx, W. H. E., Coulter, D., Craig, E. M., Reeve, A., Schalock, R. L., Snell, M. E., Spitalnik, D. M., Spreat, S., & Tassé, M. J. (2002). *Mental retardation: Definition, classification, and systems of support* (10th ed.). Washington, DC: American Association on Mental Retardation.

Massachusetts Department of Mental Retardation. (2004). *Quality assurance report for fiscal years 2002–2003.* Boston: Author.

Maturana, H. R., & Varela, F. J. (1992). *The tree of knowledge.* Boston: Shambhala.

McKeown, B., & Thomas, D. (1988). *Q methodology.* Newbury Park, CA: Sage.

Mintzberg, H. (1973). *The nature of managerial work.* New York: Harper & Row.

Mintzberg, H. (1989). The machine organization. In H. Mintzberg (Ed.), *Mintzberg on management: Inside our strange world of organizations* (pp. 173–192). New York: Free Press.

Myers, F., Ager, A., Kerr, P., & Myles, S. (1998). Outside looking in? Studies of the community integration of people with learning disabilities. *Disability and Society, 13,* 389–413.

National Committee for Quality Assurance. (2006). *The health plan employer data information set.* Washington, DC: Author.

National Core Indicators. (2005). Data brief: Factors influencing access to health care. *Core Report, 4.1.* Cambridge, MA: Human Services Research Institute.

National Institute of Mental Health. (1989). *Data standards for mental health decision support system: 1989.* Rockville, MD: Author.

National Research Council, Committee on Identifying Data Needs for Placed-Based Decision Making. (2002). *Community and quality of life: Data needs for informed decision making.* Washington, DC: National Academy Press.

Newcomer, K. E. (Ed.). (1997). *Using performance measurement to improve public and nonprofit programs*. San Francisco: Jossey-Bass.

Newman, D. L., & Brown, R. D. (1996). *Applied ethics in program evaluation*. Thousand Oaks, CA: Sage.

Newton, J. S., & Horner, R. H. (2004). Emerging trends in methods for research and evaluation of behavioral interventions. In E. Emerson, C. Hatton, T. Thompson, & T. R. Parmenter (Eds.), *The international handbook of applied research in intellectual disabilities* (pp. 495–516). West Sussex: England: John Wiley.

Nonaka, I., & Takeuchi, H. (1995). *The knowledge creating company: How Japanese companies create the dynamics of innovation*. New York: Oxford University Press.

O'Keefe, G. (1976). *Georgia O'Keefe*. New York: Viking Press.

Oxx, S. (2005, May). *Massachusetts 2002 mortality report: How are we doing in life?* Paper presented at the 21st Annual Home and Community-Based Waiver Conference, Orlando, FL.

Patton, M. Q. (1997). *Utilization-focused evaluation* (3rd ed.). Beverly Hills, CA: Sage.

Payne, S. (2005). *Using data to improve the quality of older peoples' medication use*. PowerPoint presentation at the 21st National Home and Community-Based Services Waiver Conference, Orlando, FL.

Perry, J., & Felce, D. (2005a). Correlation between subjective and objective measures of outcomes in staffed community housing. *Journal of Intellectual Disability Research, 49*(4), 278–287.

Perry, J., & Felce, D. (2005b). Factors associated with outcomes in community group homes. *American Journal on Mental Retardation, 110*(2), 121–135.

Peters, T., & Waterman, R. H. (1982). *In search of excellence: Lessons from America's best-run companies*. New York: Harper Collins.

Piaget, J. (1971). *Biology and knowledge*. Chicago: University of Chicago Press.

Pink, D. H. (2005). *A whole new mind: Moving from the information age to the conceptual age*. New York: Penguin, Riverhead.

Poston, D., Turnbull, A., Park, J., Mannan, H., Marquis, J., & Wang, M. (2003). Family quality of life: A qualitative inquiry. *Mental Retardation, 41*, 313–328.

Prouty, R. W., Smith, G., & Lakin, K.C. (2005). *Residential services for persons with developmental disabilities: Status and trends through 2004*. Minneapolis: University of Minnesota.

Putnam, R. D. (2000). *Bowling alone: The collapse and revival of American community*. New York: Simon & Schuster.

Putnam, R. D., & Feldstein, L. M. (2003). *Better together: Restoring the American community.* New York: Simon & Schuster.

Pyzdek. T. (2003). *The six sigma handbook: The complete guide for greenbelts, blackbelts, and managers at all levels.* New York: McGraw Hill.

Reger, R. K., Gustafson, L. T., DeMarie, S. M., & Mullane, J. V. (1994). Reframing the organization: Why implementing total quality is easier said than done. *Academy of Management Review, 19*(3), 565–584.

Rehabilitation Act of 1973, 29 U.S.C. § 794.

Reinders, H. (1999). The ethics of normalization. *Cambridge Quarterly of Health Care Ethics, 6,* 481–489.

Renwick, R., Brown, I., & Raphael, D. (2000). Personal-centered quality of life: Contributions from Canada to an international understanding. In K. D. Keith & R. L. Schalock (Eds.), *Cross-cultural perspectives on quality of life* (pp. 5–22). Washington, DC: American Association on Mental Retardation.

Rhode Island Division of Developmental Disabilities. (2003). *The more we know: Summary information/data from various initiatives, projects, reviews relating to systems.* Unpublished report prepared for the Rhode Island Consortium.

Robbins, S. P. (1990). *Organization theory: Structure, design, and application.* Englewood Cliffs, NJ: Prentice-Hall.

Rogers, E. M. (1995). *Diffusion of innovations* (4th ed.). New York: Free Press.

Rowe, J. E., & Taub, S. (2002). *Trend analysis of CMS regional office waiver reviews.* Unpublished paper. Available from Human Services Research Institute, Cambridge, MA.

Sandow, D. (2004). *The nature of social collaboration.* Unpublished manuscript.

Sandow, D., & Allen, A. M. (2004, February). *The nature of social collaboration.* Unpublished paper.

Sanmartin, C., Ng, E., Blackwell, D., Gentleman, J., Martinez, M., & Simile, C. (2003). *Joint Canada/United States survey of health, 2002–2003.* Ottawa, ON: Statistics, Canada; Atlanta, GA: Centers for Disease Control and Prevention.

Sante Fe Summit on Behavioral Health. (1997). *Preserving quality and value in the managed care equation: Final report.* Pittsburgh: American College of Mental Health Administrators.

Sashkin, M., & Kiser, K. J. (1993). *Putting total quality management to work: What TQM means, how to use it and how to sustain it over the long run.* San Francisco: Berrett-Koehler.

Savage, C. M. (1996). *5th generation management: Co-creating through virtual enterprising, dynamic teaming and knowledge networking.* Newton, MA: Butterworth-Heinemann.

Saxe, J. G. (1963). *The blind men and the elephant: John Godfrey Saxe's version of the famous Indian legend.* New York: Whittlesey House.

Schalock, R. L. (Ed.). (1997). *Quality of life. Vol. 2: Application to persons with disabilities.* Washington, DC: American Association on Mental Retardation.

Schalock, R. L. (2001). *Outcomes-based evaluation* (2nd ed.). New York: Kluwer

Schalock, R. L. (2004). The concept of quality of life: What we know and do not know. *Journal of Intellectual Disability Research, 48*(3), 203–216.

Schalock, R. L. (2005). Introduction and overview to the special issue. *Journal of Intellectual Disability Research, 49*(10), 695–698.

Schalock, R. L., & Bonham, G. S. (2003). Measuring outcomes and managing for results. *Evaluation and Program Planning, 26*(3), 229–235.

Schalock, R. L., Bonham, G. S., & Marchand, C. B. (2000). Consumer based quality of life assessment: A path model of perceived satisfaction. *Evaluation and Program Planning, 23*(1), 77–88.

Schalock, R. L., Brown, I., Brown, R., Cummins, R. A., Felce, D., Matikka, L., Keith, K. D., & Parmenter, T. (2002). Conceptualization, measurement, and application of quality of life for persons with intellectual disabilities: Results of an international panel of experts. *Mental Retardation, 40*(6), 457–470.

Schalock, R. L., & Felce, D. (2004). Quality of life and subjective well-being: Conceptual measurement issues. In E. Emerson, C. Hatton, T. Thompson, & T. R. Parmenter (Eds.), *International handbook of applied research in intellectual disabilities* (pp. 261–279). London: John Wiley.

Schalock, R. L., & Keith, K. D. (1993). *Quality of Life Questionnaire.* Worthington, OH: IDS.

Schalock, R. L., & Luckasson, R. (2005). *Clinical judgment.* Washington, DC: American Association on Mental Retardation.

Schalock, R. L., & Verdugo, M. A. (2002). *Handbook on quality of life for human service practitioners.* Washington, DC: American Association on Mental Retardation.

Schalock, R. L., Verdugo, M. A., Jenaro, C., Wang, M., Wehmeyer, M., Xu, J., & Lachapelle, Y. (2005). A cross-cultural study of quality of life indicators. *American Journal on Mental Retardation, 110,* 298–311.

Schein, E. (1992). *Organizational culture and leadership.* San Francisco: Jossey-Bass.

Schwartz, R., & Mayne, J. (2005). Assuring the quality of evaluation information: Theory and practice. *Evaluation and Program Planning, 28*(1), 1–14.

Seligman, A. B. (1997). *The problem of trust*. Princeton, NJ: Princeton University Press.

Senge, P. M. (1990). *The fifth discipline*. New York: Doubleday, Currency.

Smith, G., O'Keefe, I., Carpenter, L., Dota, P., & Kennedy, G. (2000). *Understanding Medicaid Home and Community Services: A primer*. Washington, DC: U.S. Department of Health & Human Services, Office of the Assistant Secretary for Planning and Evaluation.

Sparrow, S. S., Balla, D. A., & Cicchetti, D. V. (1984). *Vineland Adaptive Behavior Scales*. Circle Pines, MN: American Guidance Service.

Stacey, R. D. (1992). *Managing the unknowable: Strategic boundaries between order and chaos in organizations*. San Francisco: Jossey-Bass.

Stack, J. (1992). *The great game of business*. New York: Doubleday, Currency.

Stancliffe, R. J. (2000). Proxy respondents and quality of life. *Evaluation and Program Planning, 23*(1), 89–93.

Stancliffe, R. J., & Lakin, K. C. (2005). *Costs and outcomes of community services for people with intellectual disabilities*. Baltimore: Paul H. Brookes.

Stone, R. (1996). *The healing art of storytelling*. New York: Hyperion.

Stone, W. (2003). Bonding, bridging and linking with social capital. *Stronger Families Learning Exchange Bulletin (4)*, 13–16. [Australian Institute of Family Studies.]

Stone, W., & Hughes, J. (2000, Winter). What role for social capital in public policy? *Family Matters*, pp. 20–27.

Stone, W., & Hughes, J. (2002). Social capital: Empirical meaning and measurement validity. *Research Paper (27)*. [Australian Institute of Family Studies.]

Summers, J. A., Poston, D. J., Turnbull, A. P., Marquis, J., Hoffman, L., Manan, H., & Wang, M. (2005). Conceptualizing and measuring family quality of life. *Journal of Intellectual Disability Research, 49*(10), 777–783.

Swenson, S. (2005). Families, research, and systems change. *Mental Retardation, 43*(5), 365–368.

Tasse, M. J., Schalock, R., Thompson, J. R., & Wehmeyer, M. (2005). *Guidelines for interviewing people with disabilities: Supports Intensity Scale*. Washington, DC: American Association on Mental Retardation.

Tenner, E. (1996). *Why things bite back: Technology and the revenge of unlimited consequences*. New York: Alfred A. Knopf.

Thompson, J. R., Bryant B., Campbell, E. M., Craig, E. M., Hughes, C., Rotholz, D. A., Schalock, R. L., Silverman, W., & Tasse, M. J. (2004). *Supports Intensity Scale*. Washington, DC: American Association on Mental Retardation.

Tomer, T. F. (2003). Understanding human welfare. *Indicators (2)*3, 105–129.

Tractenberg, A. (1965). *Brooklyn Bridge: Fact and symbol*. Chicago: University of Chicago Press.

Trout, J., & Rivkin, S. (1999). *The power of simplicity: A management guide to cutting through the nonsense and doing things right*. New York: McGraw-Hill.

Turnbull, A., Brown, I., & Turnbull, H. R. III. (Eds.). (2004). *Families and people with mental retardation and quality of life: International perspectives*. Washington, DC: American Association on Mental Retardation.

Turnbull, H. R. III, Wilcox, B. L., Stowe, M. J., & Umbarger, G. T. III. (2001). Matrix of federal statutes and federal and state court decisions reflecting the core concepts of disability policy. *Journal of Disability Policy Studies, 12*(3), 144–176.

U.S. Department of Health & Human Services, Centers for Medicare & Medicaid Services. (2000). *CMS regional office protocol for conducting full reviews of state Medicaid Home and Community-Based Services Waiver Programs* (Version 1.2). Baltimore: Author.

U.S. Department of Health & Human Services, Centers for Medicare & Medicaid Services. (2002). *CMS regional office protocol for conducting full reviews of State Medicaid Home and Community-Based Services Waiver Programs*. Washington, DC: Author.

U.S. Department of Health & Human Services, Centers for Medicare & Medicaid Services. Centers for Medicare and Medicaid Services. (2003). *Workbook: Improving the quality of home and community based services and supports*. Prepared by Edmund S. Muskie School of Public Services under CMS Publication No. CMS-01-00328.

U.S. Department of Health & Human Services, Centers for Medicare & Medicaid Services. (2005a, April). *Draft application: Version 3.1 for use by states*. Baltimore: Author.

U.S. Department of Health & Human Services, Centers for Medicare & Medicaid Services. (2005b). *Quality letters* (1–9). Retrieved October 5, 2005, from https://cms.hhs.gov/medicaid/waiversqcomm.asp

U.S. Government Accounting Office. (2003). Long-term care: Federal oversight of growing Medicaid Home and Community-Based Waivers should be strengthened (GAO Publication No. 03-576). Washington, DC: Author.

U.S. Office of Management & Budget. (2002). *Program assessment rating tool (PART)*. Washington, DC: Author.

Vail, P. B. (1993). *Managing as a performing art: New ideas for a world of chaotic change.* San Francisco: Jossey-Bass.

Verdugo, M. A., Schalock, R. L., Keith, K. D., & Stancliffe, R. (2005). Quality of life and its measurement: Important principles and guidelines. *Journal of Intellectual Disability Research, 49*(10), 707–717.

Vermont Division of Developmental Services. (2005). Vermont state system of care plan for developmental services: 3-year plan. Retrieved October 5, 2005, from http://www.ddmhs.state.vt.us/docs/ds/dsSCPFy05-Fy07.pdf

Von Krogh, G., Ichijo, K., & Nonaka, I. (2000). *Enabling knowledge creation: How to unlock the mystery of tacit knowledge and release the power of innovation.* Oxford: Oxford University Press.

Waldrop, M. M. (1992). *Complexity: The emerging science at the edge of order and chaos.* New York: Touchstone.

Wheatley, M. (1994). *Leadership and the new science: Learning about organization from an orderly universe.* San Francisco: Berrett-Koehler.

Wheatley, M. J., & Kellner-Rogers, M. (1996). *A simpler way.* San Francisco: Berrett-Koehler.

Wholey, J. S. (1987). Evaluability assessment, developing program theory. In L. Bickman (Ed.), *Using program theory in evaluation: New directions for program evaluation* (pp. 60–81). San Francisco: Jossey-Bass.

Wolfensberger, W. (1992). *A brief introduction to social role valorization as a high-order concept for structuring human services* (2nd ed.). Syracuse, NY: Syracuse University, Training Institute for Human Service Planning, Leadership and Change Agency.

World Health Organization Quality of Life Work Group. (1995). The World Health Organization Quality of Life Assessment (WHOQOL): Position paper from the World Health Organization. *Social Science Medicine, 41*(10), 1403–1409.

Wyatt v. Stickney, 105 F. Supp. 1234 (M.D. Ala. 2000).

Zuboff, S. (1988). *In the age of the smart machine: The future of work and power.* New York: Basic Books.

Subject Index

Accountability
  changing approaches to, 16
  pressure for, 103-104
Aggregating individual data
  See: Reporting issues; comparison
    issues
Ask Me! Project (Maryland), 41-43

Basic Assurances, 74
Benchmarks, 81, 124
Bridging Organizations, 52-53

Centers for Medicare and Medicaid
    Services (CMS)
  Government Accounting Office
    (GAO) critique, 105
  interim procedural guidance and
    new waiver application, 106
  quality framework, 105
  relation to National Core
    Indicators, 131-132
Community life context, 161-165
Comparison issues, 39-40, 81-82, 124
Consumers
  as key players, 173-174
  as quality of life surveyors, 42
Core domains and indicators
  See: QOL domains: QOL
    indicators
Council on Quality and Leadership
  national personal outcome
    measures data base, 79-85
  description and history, 74-75

personal outcome measures, 75-78
  research and development, 78-79
Culture, 56-62
  See also: Management of personal
    outcomes

Developmental disabilities
  definition, xii
Direct support professionals, 54, 57

Emerging challenges and opportunities
  See: Consumers as key players;
    Organizations redefining their
    role; Quality of life
  assessment and feedback; quality
    of life as a change agent;
    quality improvement
Evaluation and reporting standards, 107
Evaluation theory, 12

Government Performance and
  Reporting Act of 1993, 103

Intellectual disabilities
  definition, xii
Information collection process
  ethical principles, 32-33
  guidelines, 32-33
  principles involved in, 32-34
  two-components, 30
Innovation, 71-72

Leadership
  leadership themes, 168
  See also: Management of personal
    outcomes

Management of personal outcomes
  culture, 59-62
  execution, 56-59
  leadership, 64-69
  strategy, 51-56, 176-177
  structure, 62-64
Measurement
  challenges and potential resistance,
    40-41
  of quality outcomes: measurement
    principles, 31-32
  of personal outcomes
    interviewing techniques, 34
    procedural issues, 34-41
    use of proxies, 34-35, 37
    value of measuring, 30
  See also: Information collection
    process; Psychometric standards
Mental models
  analysis vs. synthesis, 152-153
  mechanistic vs. organic
    organizations, 151-152
  planned vs. self-organizing
    emergent systems, 153-155
  reductionism vs. systems thinking,
    150-151
  tacit vs. explicit knowledge, 156-
    157
  thinking vs. doing, 155-156
Methodological pluralism, 12

National Core Indicators Project, 110-
    127
  indicators, 110, 114-116

Organizations
  managing for change, 48-49
  redefining their roles, 174-176
Outcomes
  See: Personal outcomes;
    Performance indicators

Participatory action research, 41-43
Performance indicators
  definition, xii
  development of, 111-112
  personal outcome measures purpose
    of, 112-113
  See also: Systems-level performance
    indicators
Person-centered planning, 87-88
Personal outcomes
  definition, xi, 11-12
  guidelines for their use, 7
  managing for, 75-79, 165-167
  measures and associated quality
    indicators, 21-25, 73
  predictors of, 9-11
  principles, 88-89
  values, 30
  See also: Evaluation theory;
    information collection process;
    management of personal
    outcomes; measurement
Program evaluation theory, 12
Program logic models, 10

Proxies
    effectiveness, 37
    use of, 34-35
Psychometric standards, 35-39, 118-119

Quality assurance, 74
Quality domains
    associated indicators, 9, 20-25
    definition, xii
    literature review of, 19-25
Quality improvement
    a community life context for quality of life, 161-165
    approaches to, 89-91
    as a continuous process, 58, 133, 177-180
    definition, xii, 74
    examples of, 133-139
    managing for personal outcomes, 75-79, 165-167
    See: Quality strategies; Social capital
Quality indicators
    context, 7-8, 16-17
    criteria for selecting, 26-28
    definition, xii
    examples, 20-25
    use of, 16-19
Quality of life
    application principles, 6, 144-145, 169
    as a change agent, 171-172
    assessment and feedback to stakeholders, 172-173
    concept, 1, 3

conceptualization principles, 6, 169
definition, 74
domains
    See: Quality domains
evolution of the concept, 4-6
history of, 4
indicators
    See: Quality indicators
measurement principles, 6, 31-32, 144, 169
multidimensionality of, 6
predictors of quality of life outcomes, 9-11
programmatic emphasis, 85-91, 98-99
subjective and objective aspects of, 8-9
uses of, 1
Quality strategies
    psychometric standards, 35-39, 118-119
    proxies and use of, 34-35
    effectiveness of, 37
    See: Mental models; Quality improvement; Reframing quality
Quality system, 72-73

Reframing quality, 158
Reporting issues, 39

Service delivery system
    changes in, 99-103
Social capital, 158-161
Social indicators, 11
Social policy, 95-100

Stories, 54

Strategy, 50-55

Systems change, 100-102

Systems-level performance indicators
    data collection tools, 119
    emerging practices and challenges,
        130, 139-142
    evolution, 100-104
    examples, 114-115, 124-127
    purpose, 97-98
    quality of life emphasis, 98-99
    rationale for their use, 122-124
    selection criteria, 116
    selection of, 113, 122-123

Transitions, 170

Utilization-focused evaluation, 12

Printed in the United States
81190LV00003B/1-136

9 780940 898967